Reclaim

Your Life

Reclaim Your Life

A Self-Therapy Guide to Overcoming Addiction
to Masturbation and Pornography

Olivier Moreau

Title: Reclaim Your Life
Subtitle: A Self-Therapy Guide to Overcoming Addiction to Masturbation
and Pornography
Author: Olivier Moreau

ISBN 9798301355226

Edition I, Montreal, 2024

Introduction

In the modern digital era, where screens dominate our lives, an alarming number of individuals find themselves ensnared by the grips of pornography and compulsive masturbation. These behaviors, once considered taboo or dismissed as minor indulgences, have escalated into a serious public health concern. With the internet offering instant and unlimited access to explicit content, the line between occasional use and dependency has become increasingly blurred. For many, this dependency leads to a cascade of negative effects—emotional isolation, strained relationships, diminished self-esteem, and even impacts on professional and academic performance.

This book, **"Reclaim Your Life: A Self-Therapy Guide to Overcoming Addiction to Masturbation and Pornography,"** aims to address this sensitive yet pressing issue with compassion, expertise, and practical solutions. The goal is not to judge but to provide a roadmap for those ready to confront these challenges head-on. Whether you've been struggling for years or have recently recognized patterns of behavior you'd like to change, this guide offers a path toward healing, self-control, and a renewed sense of purpose.

Why This Book Matters

Addiction to pornography and compulsive masturbation often thrives in silence and secrecy. Those affected may feel too embarrassed to seek help or may downplay the severity of their situation. Yet, the consequences of unchecked addiction can ripple through every facet of life, eroding mental health, distorting perceptions of intimacy, and fostering feelings of guilt and shame. This guide breaks the silence by fostering an open, nonjudgmental conversation about the realities of this addiction and offering actionable steps for recovery.

The uniqueness of this book lies in its approach. It is a self-therapy guide, designed to empower you to take charge of your recovery. While professional therapy and support groups can be invaluable, not everyone has access to these resources or feels ready to take that step. Self-therapy offers a starting point—an opportunity to understand the roots of your addiction, develop strategies for managing triggers, and rebuild your life at your own pace.

Understanding the Problem

At its core, addiction to pornography and masturbation isn't just about the behavior itself; it's about what drives it. Often, these behaviors serve as coping mechanisms for deeper emotional struggles—stress, loneliness, anxiety, or even boredom. Over time, they can become entrenched habits, rewiring the brain to seek instant gratification at the expense of long-term well-being.

It's essential to recognize that this addiction is not a moral failing or a lack of willpower. It's a complex interplay of biology, psychology, and environmental factors. Understanding this complexity is the first step toward recovery. This book will guide you through that understanding, providing insights into how addiction works, why it persists, and how you can break free.

Who This Book Is For

This guide is for anyone who feels trapped by compulsive behaviors related to pornography and masturbation. Whether you're a teenager grappling with newfound urges, an adult feeling the strain on your relationships, or someone in any stage of life seeking to regain control, this book offers something for you. It's also a resource for those supporting loved ones facing these challenges, providing them with tools to understand and assist without judgment.

The Power of Self-Therapy

Self-therapy is an empowering approach that places the tools for recovery in your hands. It's about learning to be honest with yourself, setting realistic goals, and cultivating habits that support long-term change. Through self-reflection, mindfulness, and practical exercises, you can identify the triggers and thought patterns that sustain your addiction and replace them with healthier alternatives.

This book doesn't promise a quick fix. Overcoming addiction is a journey that requires patience, perseverance, and self-compassion. However, it does promise that change is possible. With commitment and the right tools, you can reclaim your life, rediscover your sense of self-worth, and build a future free from the constraints of addiction.

How to Use This Guide

Each chapter of this book is designed to address a specific aspect of addiction and recovery. You'll begin by understanding the science behind addiction, exploring its emotional and psychological impacts, and identifying the signs that indicate a problem. From there, you'll delve into practical strategies for breaking the cycle, building resilience, and nurturing a healthier relationship with yourself and others.

It's important to approach this journey with an open mind and a willingness to engage fully with the process. Some exercises may feel challenging or uncomfortable, but they are essential steps toward growth and healing. Remember, recovery is not about perfection; it's about progress.

You don't have to read this book from cover to cover in one sitting. Instead, take it at your own pace, revisiting chapters as needed and applying the strategies in your daily life. Think of it as a companion on your journey—a source of guidance, encouragement, and practical advice.

A Journey Toward Freedom and Self-Respect

Addiction can often make you feel powerless, as though you've lost control of your choices and your life. But the truth is, you have the strength within you to change. This book is here to help you harness that strength, guiding you toward a life of freedom, self-respect, and authentic connection.

By choosing to address your addiction, you are taking the first and most important step toward reclaiming your life. It's not an easy journey, but it's one worth taking. And as you work through the chapters of this guide, you'll discover not only how to overcome your addiction but also how to build a life filled with meaning, joy, and self-compassion.

Welcome to the first step of your transformation. Let's begin.

Why This Book Matters

In a world increasingly dominated by digital technology, the challenges posed by pornography and compulsive masturbation are more prevalent than ever before. The accessibility of explicit content has transformed what was once considered a private matter into a widespread issue, affecting millions globally. This book, *Reclaim Your Life: A Self-Therapy Guide to Overcoming Addiction to Masturbation and Pornography,* addresses this issue head-on, not with judgment or shame, but with understanding and practical tools for recovery.

Pornography addiction often operates in silence. Many individuals feel trapped in a cycle of compulsive behavior, struggling to reconcile their actions with their values and aspirations. For some, the stigma surrounding this topic prevents them from seeking help, leaving them isolated and overwhelmed. Despite being a pervasive issue, it is rarely discussed openly, and those who suffer may feel as though they are alone in their struggles. This silence can have profound consequences. Addiction to pornography and masturbation impacts mental health, relationships, self-esteem, and even physical well-being. Yet, because of the nature of the issue, those affected often endure their battles without support, perpetuating a cycle of guilt and helplessness. This book seeks to break that silence. By addressing these challenges openly and empathetically, it creates a space where individuals can confront their struggles without fear of judgment.

Unlike many resources that either sensationalize the issue or approach it from an overly clinical perspective, this book aims to bridge the gap by combining expert knowledge with accessible, actionable advice. It recognizes that not everyone has access to therapy or support groups, and not everyone feels ready to discuss their struggles with others. That's where self-therapy becomes invaluable. Self-therapy empowers individuals to take control of their recovery. It provides the tools needed to understand the root causes of addiction, identify triggers, and develop strategies for change. This book equips readers with these tools, offering a step-by-step approach to overcoming addiction in a way that is manageable and tailored to their unique circumstances.

One of the defining features of this book is its holistic approach. Addiction is rarely a standalone issue; it often intertwines with other aspects of life, such as emotional well-being, relationships, and self-image. Therefore, recovery requires more than just breaking the habit—it involves rebuilding a life that is fulfilling and free from the constraints of addiction. This guide delves into every facet of the recovery process, from understanding the psychological and biological mechanisms of addiction to cultivating healthier habits and relationships. By addressing the issue from multiple angles, it ensures that readers not only overcome their addiction but also gain the tools to thrive in all areas of life.

Another critical aspect of this book is its commitment to reducing the stigma surrounding pornography and masturbation addiction. These issues are often accompanied by feelings of shame and self-judgment, which can hinder the recovery process. This book approaches the topic with empathy, helping readers understand that addiction is not a moral failing but a challenge that can be addressed with the right strategies and support. By normalizing the conversation, the book encourages readers to approach their recovery with self-compassion rather than self-condemnation. It fosters a sense of hope, reminding them that they are not alone in their struggles and that change is possible.

At its core, this book is about empowerment. It acknowledges the difficulties of addiction while emphasizing the potential for growth and transformation. Recovery is not just about giving something up; it's about reclaiming your life, rediscovering your self-worth, and building a future aligned with your values and aspirations. For anyone feeling trapped by compulsive behaviors, this book serves as a beacon of hope. It offers a roadmap for change, guiding readers through the process of understanding their addiction, breaking free from its grip, and creating a life of freedom and fulfillment.

The journey of recovery can be daunting, but it is also profoundly rewarding. This book exists to remind readers that no matter how deep their struggles, there is always a way forward. With patience, determination, and the right tools, it is possible to overcome addiction and build a life that is rich in meaning and joy. *Reclaim Your Life* is more than just a guide—it's an invitation to take the first step toward transformation. It's a reminder that while addiction may feel overwhelming, it does not define you.

Understanding the Problem: Addiction to Pornography and Masturbation

Addiction to pornography and masturbation is a multifaceted issue that extends far beyond simple habits or occasional indulgences. It is a complex interplay of psychological, emotional, and biological factors that can lead individuals into a cycle of dependency. Understanding this problem requires an exploration of how addiction forms, why it persists, and the profound effects it has on various aspects of life. By grasping the underlying mechanisms, individuals can begin to untangle themselves from its grip and move toward recovery with clarity and purpose.

At its core, addiction is a condition in which the brain's reward system is hijacked. Normally, pleasurable activities such as eating, exercising, or connecting with others release dopamine, a neurotransmitter that reinforces positive behaviors and motivates repetition. However, pornography and compulsive masturbation exploit this system in unnatural ways. The highly stimulating and novel content available online triggers massive surges of dopamine, far exceeding what is typically experienced in daily life. Over time, the brain adapts by reducing its sensitivity to dopamine, requiring more intense stimulation to achieve the same effect. This phenomenon, known as desensitization, lies at the heart of addiction.

Compounding this is the cycle of reinforcement that addiction creates. Pornography and masturbation often serve as coping mechanisms for stress, boredom, loneliness, or other uncomfortable emotions. They provide an immediate, albeit temporary, escape from reality, offering a sense of comfort and distraction. However, the relief they bring is short-lived and often followed by feelings of guilt, shame, or dissatisfaction. These negative emotions, in turn, drive individuals to seek out the same behaviors again, perpetuating a loop that becomes increasingly difficult to break.

The digital age has amplified the accessibility and prevalence of pornography to an unprecedented degree. With smartphones, tablets, and computers, explicit content is just a click away, available 24/7 and often free of charge. The ease of access eliminates traditional barriers such as social stigma or physical effort, making it easier than ever to indulge in these behaviors without external scrutiny. Furthermore, the endless variety of material available online provides a constant stream of novelty, keeping users engaged and reinforcing addictive tendencies.

Beyond its effects on the brain, addiction to pornography and masturbation impacts nearly every facet of life. Emotionally, it can lead to feelings of isolation and a diminished sense of self-worth. Many individuals caught in the cycle of addiction feel ashamed or embarrassed, believing they lack the willpower to stop. This self-perception can erode their confidence and create a sense of hopelessness. Socially, addiction can interfere with relationships, leading to misunderstandings, conflicts, or even breakdowns in trust. Partners may feel neglected, hurt, or inadequate, while the individual struggling with addiction may withdraw emotionally, further straining the bond.

From a physical perspective, excessive masturbation can sometimes lead to issues such as fatigue, diminished sexual sensitivity, or even physical discomfort. These physical consequences, while often reversible, can compound the emotional toll of addiction, reinforcing feelings of inadequacy or frustration. Academically or professionally, addiction can detract from focus, productivity, and overall performance. Time spent engaging in compulsive behaviors is time taken away from personal growth, relationships, or career advancement, leading to a sense of stagnation.

Cultural and societal attitudes toward pornography and masturbation further complicate the issue. While these behaviors are often normalized or even celebrated in some contexts, they are also stigmatized or dismissed in others. This dichotomy can leave individuals feeling confused or conflicted about their actions, making it harder to recognize when a problem exists. The normalization of explicit content, especially in mainstream media, can desensitize individuals to its potential harms, while stigma discourages open discussion or seeking help.

Recognizing addiction is the first step toward recovery. For many, this recognition comes when the negative effects of their behavior become undeniable—strained relationships, declining mental health, or a pervasive sense of dissatisfaction with life. It is essential to understand that addiction is not a moral failing or a sign of weakness but a condition rooted in the brain's wiring and environmental influences. Approaching it with this perspective allows individuals to move forward with compassion for themselves and a willingness to take the necessary steps toward change.

Breaking free from addiction begins with identifying the triggers and patterns that sustain it. These triggers can vary widely, from stress and loneliness to specific environments or routines. Understanding what drives the behavior provides the foundation for developing strategies to counteract it. Equally important is addressing the underlying emotional needs that addiction often masks. Learning to manage stress, build meaningful connections, and engage in fulfilling activities can help replace destructive habits with positive ones.

Addiction to pornography and masturbation is a challenging issue, but it is also one that can be overcome. By understanding its mechanisms and recognizing its effects, individuals can take the first steps toward reclaiming their lives. The journey requires patience, self-reflection, and a commitment to change, but the rewards—a renewed sense of freedom, self-respect, and connection—are well worth the effort. This book aims to provide the tools, guidance, and support needed to navigate this path and emerge stronger, healthier, and more fulfilled.

Who This Book Is For

This book is for anyone who feels trapped in the cycle of compulsive pornography use and masturbation. It is for those who have recognized that these behaviors are no longer serving their lives in a positive way and are instead causing distress, dissatisfaction, or harm. Whether you are just beginning to notice the negative effects of these habits or have been struggling with them for years, this guide is designed to meet you where you are and provide practical, actionable steps toward recovery.

It is not uncommon to feel isolated or unique in this struggle, but you are far from alone. Millions of people around the world face similar challenges, often in silence and secrecy. This book speaks to anyone who feels ashamed, confused, or overwhelmed by their behavior, offering a safe space to explore these feelings without judgment. If you have ever wondered whether your relationship with pornography or masturbation is healthy or questioned whether you are in control of these habits, this book is for you. It is a resource for anyone ready to take an honest look at their behavior and make meaningful changes to reclaim their life.

This guide is also for those who may not yet identify as addicted but are curious about how these behaviors affect their mental, emotional, and physical well-being. It can help you develop awareness and understanding before these habits escalate into more significant issues. By addressing the underlying factors early, you can prevent the patterns of compulsive behavior from taking root.

For individuals who feel a sense of helplessness or defeat, this book offers hope. Recovery can seem like an insurmountable challenge, especially when past attempts to change have failed. This guide acknowledges the setbacks and struggles that are a natural part of the process and provides tools to help you persevere. It reminds you that change is not about perfection but progress, and it encourages self-compassion every step of the way.

This book is also a valuable resource for those who have already sought professional help or are participating in a support group but want additional tools to aid their journey. It complements external resources by offering a structured, self-guided approach that you can tailor to your unique needs and circumstances. It is designed to empower you to take control of your recovery and build the skills necessary for lasting change.

Beyond those directly struggling with addiction, this book is for partners, friends, and family members who want to better understand the challenges their loved ones are facing. Addiction to pornography and masturbation can strain relationships, leading to feelings of betrayal, confusion, or hurt. This guide provides insights into the nature of these struggles, helping loved ones approach the situation with empathy and support rather than judgment or frustration. Understanding the problem is the first step toward fostering healthy communication and rebuilding trust.

Finally, this book is for anyone who believes in the possibility of change. You may have doubts, fears, or uncertainties about whether recovery is attainable, and that is completely normal. This guide is here to show you that transformation is not only possible but within your reach. It is not about erasing the past or punishing yourself for mistakes but about building a future rooted in self-respect, freedom, and fulfillment.

No matter your age, background, or personal circumstances, this book is written with you in mind. It recognizes the diversity of experiences and challenges that come with addiction and offers guidance that is flexible and adaptable to your situation. Whether you are reading this book in private, seeking a quiet moment of reflection, or using it as a companion on a longer journey, know that you are taking a powerful step forward.

If you are ready to take control of your life and confront these challenges with courage and determination, this book is for you. It is an invitation to embark on a journey of self-discovery and growth, to learn new ways of thinking and living, and to reclaim the sense of purpose and joy that addiction may have taken from you. You are not alone in this, and the tools and insights within these pages are here to guide and support you every step of the way.

The Power of Self-Therapy

The power of self-therapy lies in its ability to empower individuals to take control of their recovery journey. Unlike traditional therapy, which often involves guidance from a professional, self-therapy puts the tools and techniques directly into your hands. It allows you to address the roots of your addiction, develop coping mechanisms, and rebuild your life at a pace and in a manner that feels right for you. This approach recognizes that not everyone has access to therapy or feels comfortable seeking help from others, making it an accessible and effective option for many.

Self-therapy is not about isolating yourself or believing you can solve everything alone. Instead, it is about cultivating self-awareness and learning to be your own ally in the recovery process. At its core, self-therapy is a commitment to understanding yourself better—your thoughts, emotions, triggers, and behaviors—and using that understanding to create meaningful change. It requires honesty, patience, and a willingness to face uncomfortable truths, but it also provides the tools to transform those truths into opportunities for growth.

One of the greatest strengths of self-therapy is its flexibility. Every individual's journey with addiction is unique, shaped by personal experiences, challenges, and aspirations. Self-therapy allows you to tailor your recovery plan to your specific needs, focusing on the strategies and techniques that resonate most with you. This adaptability ensures that your approach feels relevant and sustainable, increasing the likelihood of long-term success.

Another significant advantage of self-therapy is the sense of empowerment it fosters. Addiction often leaves individuals feeling powerless, as though their choices are no longer their own. Self-therapy challenges this narrative by showing that you have the capacity to take back control. Through consistent effort and self-reflection, you can dismantle the patterns that sustain your addiction and replace them with healthier, more fulfilling habits. This process is not easy, but it is deeply rewarding, as it allows you to reclaim your agency and rebuild your life on your own terms.

Self-therapy also emphasizes the importance of self-compassion. Addiction is often accompanied by feelings of shame and self-judgment, which can undermine recovery efforts. By approaching your journey with kindness and understanding, you create a foundation for healing that is rooted in acceptance rather than punishment. Self-compassion allows you to acknowledge your mistakes without letting them define you, creating space for growth and transformation.

A key element of self-therapy is the development of practical skills to manage triggers and cravings. These triggers, whether emotional, environmental, or situational, are the cues that drive addictive behaviors. Self-therapy teaches you to identify and understand these triggers, equipping you with strategies to respond to them in healthier ways. This might involve mindfulness practices to ground yourself in the present moment, relaxation techniques to manage stress, or cognitive reframing to challenge negative thought patterns.

Another focus of self-therapy is rebuilding your sense of self-worth. Addiction can erode your confidence and leave you feeling disconnected from your values and aspirations. Through self-reflection and intentional action, self-therapy helps you reconnect with what truly matters to you. It encourages you to set goals that align with your values and take steps toward achieving them, no matter how small those steps may be. Each achievement, no matter how modest, reinforces your belief in your ability to change and grow.

Self-therapy also highlights the importance of building a support system, even if your primary work is done independently. While this guide provides tools for self-directed recovery, it does not discount the value of meaningful connections with others. Whether it's sharing your journey with a trusted friend, seeking guidance from a mentor, or joining an online community, having a support network can provide encouragement, accountability, and perspective.

It's important to note that self-therapy is not a replacement for professional help when it's needed. Some individuals may find that their addiction is deeply entrenched or accompanied by other challenges, such as depression or anxiety, that require specialized care. In these cases, self-therapy can be a complementary tool, enhancing the work you do with a therapist or other professional.

The power of self-therapy ultimately lies in its ability to foster independence and resilience. It encourages you to take ownership of your recovery and to view challenges as opportunities for growth rather than obstacles. It reminds you that while the journey may be difficult, it is also a chance to rediscover your strength, rebuild your confidence, and create a life that aligns with your values and aspirations.

Through self-therapy, you can move beyond the limitations of addiction and step into a life of greater freedom, self-respect, and fulfillment. This process requires dedication and perseverance, but it also offers the profound reward of knowing that you are actively shaping your future. By embracing the principles and practices of self-therapy, you are taking a powerful step toward reclaiming your life and realizing your full potential.

How to Use This Guide

This guide is designed to be your companion on the journey toward breaking free from addiction to pornography and masturbation. It is both a resource and a roadmap, offering insights, tools, and exercises that you can use to understand and address the challenges you face. Recovery is not a linear process, and this guide respects that by allowing you to engage with its content in a way that suits your individual needs and pace. Here is how you can make the most of this guide as you embark on the path to reclaiming your life.

First, approach this guide with an open mind and a willingness to engage honestly with its content. Recovery requires confronting uncomfortable truths and stepping out of your comfort zone, but it also offers the chance for profound growth and transformation. By reading this book, you have already taken the first and most important step— acknowledging that change is needed and possible. The pages that follow are designed to support you in that process, providing practical strategies and compassionate guidance every step of the way.

This guide is structured to take you through a comprehensive journey of recovery. It begins by helping you understand the nature of addiction, including the psychological, emotional, and biological factors that contribute to it. This foundational knowledge is crucial because it allows you to recognize that your struggle is not a personal failing but a challenge rooted in complex, interconnected causes. Understanding these causes will empower you to address them effectively and with greater self-compassion.

As you move through the chapters, you will find a variety of tools and techniques for managing triggers, developing healthier habits, and rebuilding your sense of self-worth. Each chapter builds on the last, creating a cohesive framework for recovery that you can adapt to your unique circumstances. While the book is designed to be read sequentially, you are encouraged to revisit sections that resonate with you or focus on areas where you feel you need the most support. This guide is not a rigid program but a flexible resource that you can tailor to your own journey.

The exercises and strategies in this guide are practical and actionable, meant to be applied in your daily life. As you read, take the time to reflect on how each concept relates to your own experiences. Journaling can be a helpful way to document your thoughts, track your progress, and deepen your understanding of the material. Recovery is as much about self-discovery as it is about breaking habits, and engaging actively with this guide will help you uncover insights that can transform your approach to life.

One of the key principles of this guide is self-compassion. Addiction often comes with feelings of shame, guilt, or frustration, which can create barriers to recovery. This book encourages you to approach your journey with kindness and patience. Mistakes and setbacks are natural parts of the process, and they do not define your progress or your worth. By treating yourself with compassion, you create a supportive environment for growth and healing.

While this guide focuses on self-therapy, it acknowledges the value of seeking additional support when needed. You may find it helpful to share your journey with a trusted friend, partner, or support group. Connecting with others who understand or empathize with your experience can provide encouragement, accountability, and perspective. This guide complements such connections by equipping you with tools for self-reflection and personal growth, enhancing the work you do with others.

Recovery is not about achieving perfection but about making progress. This guide is here to help you set realistic goals, celebrate your successes, and learn from your challenges. As you implement the strategies and exercises, remember that small, consistent steps often lead to the most meaningful changes. Give yourself permission to grow at your own pace and to redefine what success looks like for you.

Finally, this guide is a reminder that you are not alone. Addiction can make you feel isolated, as though no one else understands what you are going through. But the truth is, many people face similar struggles, and there is hope and help available. By using this guide, you are taking a courageous step toward reclaiming your life and building a future free from the constraints of addiction. This journey may be challenging, but it is also deeply rewarding, offering the chance to rediscover your strength, reconnect with your values, and create a life of fulfillment and freedom.

As you navigate this guide, keep in mind that recovery is not just about stopping a behavior but about creating a life that aligns with your aspirations and values. This guide is here to support you in that journey, providing the tools and insights you need to move forward with confidence and hope. Take it one step at a time, and trust in your ability to create the change you seek.

A Journey Toward Freedom and Self-Respect

The journey toward freedom and self-respect begins with a single decision: the choice to confront the patterns and behaviors that no longer serve you and to seek a life aligned with your true values and aspirations. It is not an easy path, but it is one filled with potential, growth, and profound transformation. For those struggling with addiction to pornography and masturbation, this journey represents more than just breaking free from compulsive behaviors—it is about rediscovering yourself, rebuilding your sense of worth, and reclaiming control over your life.

Freedom from addiction is not merely the absence of a habit. It is a state of being in which you are no longer controlled by urges, triggers, or cravings. It is the ability to make choices that reflect your authentic self, unencumbered by the grip of compulsive behavior. Achieving this freedom requires courage, persistence, and a willingness to face discomfort, but the rewards are immeasurable. It is a journey of liberation, where each step forward reinforces your capacity to create a life of purpose and fulfillment.

Self-respect is one of the most significant gifts of recovery. Addiction often erodes our self-image, leaving behind feelings of guilt, shame, and inadequacy. These emotions can create a cycle of negativity, where the more we struggle, the worse we feel about ourselves, and the harder it becomes to make positive changes. Breaking free from this cycle is a powerful act of self-love. It is a declaration that you are worthy of happiness, health, and a future unburdened by addiction.

As you embark on this journey, it is important to acknowledge that progress is not linear. There will be challenges, setbacks, and moments of doubt. These are not signs of failure but opportunities to learn and grow. Every step you take, no matter how small, is a step toward reclaiming your freedom and building a foundation of self-respect. Recovery is a process, and it requires patience and persistence. Be gentle with yourself as you navigate this path, and remember that each effort brings you closer to your goals.

The path to freedom and self-respect begins with awareness. Recognizing the ways in which addiction has affected your life—your relationships, your mental health, your sense of self—is the first step in breaking its hold. This awareness allows you to see the impact of your choices and empowers you to make new ones. It is not about dwelling on the past or blaming yourself for your struggles. Instead, it is about taking responsibility for your future and embracing the possibility of change.

Once you have committed to this journey, it becomes a process of building new habits, perspectives, and strategies that support your recovery. These may include understanding your triggers and learning how to respond to them, cultivating healthier coping mechanisms, and finding new ways to fulfill the emotional needs that addiction once masked. Each of these steps brings you closer to the person you want to be—someone who is in control of their life, confident in their choices, and aligned with their values.

Freedom and self-respect are deeply intertwined. As you free yourself from the grip of addiction, you begin to rebuild your sense of self-worth. This renewed respect for yourself is not only a source of motivation but also a foundation for sustaining your recovery. When you value yourself, you are less likely to engage in behaviors that undermine your well-being, and you are more inclined to pursue goals and relationships that enrich your life.

This journey is also an opportunity to reconnect with the things that bring you joy and meaning. Addiction often narrows our focus, making it difficult to see beyond the immediate gratification it offers. Recovery opens the door to a broader perspective, where you can rediscover your passions, nurture your relationships, and explore new possibilities for growth and fulfillment. It is a chance to rebuild your life in a way that reflects your true self and supports your long-term happiness.

As you move forward, remember that you are not alone. Many others have walked this path and emerged stronger, healthier, and more fulfilled. Their stories are a testament to the power of resilience and the potential for transformation. By choosing to embark on this journey, you are joining a community of individuals who have faced similar challenges and overcome them. You are not defined by your addiction but by your determination to overcome it and create a life of freedom and self-respect.

This book is your companion on this journey, offering insights, tools, and encouragement to guide you along the way. It is here to remind you that change is possible, that you have the strength within you to overcome addiction, and that a life of freedom and self-respect is within your reach. Each step you take brings you closer to reclaiming your life, and with each step, you are building a future filled with possibility, purpose, and fulfillment. This is your journey, and it is one worth taking.

Spis treści

Chapter 1:
Understanding Addiction

Addiction is a complex and multifaceted condition that extends beyond mere habit or routine. It involves deeply rooted psychological, emotional, and biological mechanisms that create a powerful cycle of dependency. Understanding addiction, particularly addiction to pornography and masturbation, requires an exploration of how it develops, why it persists, and the profound impact it has on the mind and body. By shedding light on these dynamics, you can gain the clarity needed to take meaningful steps toward recovery.

At its core, addiction is a condition of the brain's reward system. Normally, this system is designed to reinforce behaviors that are essential for survival, such as eating, socializing, and procreation. When you engage in these activities, your brain releases dopamine, a neurotransmitter that creates feelings of pleasure and satisfaction. This reinforcement encourages you to repeat these behaviors, ensuring that your needs are met. However, addictive behaviors, such as compulsive pornography use and masturbation, exploit this system in unnatural ways. They deliver intense and repeated surges of dopamine that far exceed the levels generated by natural rewards. Over time, this overstimulation causes your brain to adapt by reducing its sensitivity to dopamine, a process known as desensitization. As a result, you may find yourself needing more frequent or extreme stimulation to achieve the same level of pleasure, creating a vicious cycle of dependency.

The cycle of addiction is further reinforced by the brain's habit-forming structures. Each time you engage in a behavior, neural pathways associated with that behavior are strengthened. This is especially true for repetitive actions like viewing pornography or masturbating, where the patterns of seeking, engaging, and experiencing pleasure become deeply ingrained. These pathways can become so dominant that they override other desires or priorities, making it difficult to resist urges even when you recognize their negative consequences.

Addiction to pornography and masturbation often serves as a coping mechanism for emotional or psychological distress. Stress, loneliness, boredom, anxiety, and even feelings of inadequacy can trigger these behaviors, offering a temporary escape from discomfort. The problem is that the relief provided by these actions is short-lived and superficial. Instead of addressing the root causes of these emotions, addiction creates a cycle of avoidance that leaves underlying issues unresolved. Over time, this can lead to a dependency on these behaviors as a primary means of managing stress or negative emotions, further entrenching the cycle of addiction.

Another critical aspect of addiction is its ability to distort your perception of reality. Pornography, in particular, presents an exaggerated and often unrealistic portrayal of intimacy and relationships. Regular consumption of such content can warp your expectations of real-life connections, leading to dissatisfaction, disconnection, and challenges in forming or maintaining healthy relationships. Masturbation, when driven by compulsion, can further isolate you from others, reinforcing feelings of loneliness and reducing opportunities for genuine intimacy.

The accessibility and prevalence of pornography in the digital age have amplified the challenges associated with this form of addiction. With high-speed internet and mobile devices, explicit content is readily available at any time and from virtually anywhere. The anonymity provided by these platforms makes it easy to engage in these behaviors without external scrutiny, reducing the barriers to consumption and increasing the risk of compulsive use. The sheer variety and novelty of content available online also contribute to the addictive nature of pornography. Novelty is a powerful stimulant for the brain, and the constant stream of new material keeps users engaged, reinforcing the cycle of addiction.

The consequences of addiction to pornography and masturbation are far-reaching. On an emotional level, these behaviors can lead to feelings of guilt, shame, and low self-esteem. You may feel as though you have lost control over your actions, which can erode your confidence and create a sense of helplessness. Socially, addiction can strain relationships, causing misunderstandings, conflicts, and a breakdown of trust. Partners may feel neglected, betrayed, or inadequate, while individuals struggling with addiction may withdraw emotionally, further exacerbating relational challenges.

From a physical perspective, excessive masturbation can sometimes lead to issues such as fatigue, decreased sensitivity, or physical discomfort. These effects, while often reversible, can compound the emotional toll of addiction. Additionally, the time and energy devoted to these behaviors can detract from personal goals, professional achievements, and meaningful connections, creating a sense of stagnation or unfulfilled potential.

Understanding addiction also requires recognizing its psychological impact. The repetitive nature of these behaviors can create a sense of dependency that undermines your sense of autonomy. You may feel as though your actions are no longer under your control, which can be both frustrating and demoralizing. This perception of powerlessness is a hallmark of addiction and underscores the importance of reclaiming your agency through self-awareness and intentional action.

Recovery begins with acknowledging the presence of addiction and understanding its mechanisms. It is not about blaming yourself or viewing your behavior as a moral failing but about recognizing the patterns and triggers that sustain your dependency. This awareness is the first step toward breaking free from the cycle of addiction and building a life that aligns with your values and aspirations.

Addiction is not an identity; it is a challenge—one that you have the strength and capacity to overcome. By understanding how addiction affects your brain, emotions, and behaviors, you can begin to unravel its hold and take the first steps toward recovery. The journey requires patience, persistence, and self-compassion, but it also offers the opportunity for profound growth and transformation. As you move forward, remember that recovery is not about perfection but progress. Each step you take brings you closer to reclaiming your freedom and rediscovering your true self.

1.1. What Is Addiction?

Addiction is a term that is often misunderstood, associated solely with substances like drugs or alcohol. However, addiction is not limited to chemical dependencies; it also encompasses behaviors that become compulsive and harmful over time. Understanding what addiction truly is forms the foundation for overcoming it. Addiction to pornography and masturbation is a prime example of behavioral addiction—one rooted in patterns of actions and reinforced by psychological and physiological mechanisms.

At its essence, addiction is a condition characterized by the inability to stop engaging in a behavior or using a substance despite its negative consequences. It is driven by a complex interplay of the brain's reward system, emotional needs, and environmental factors. For many, addiction begins as a way to seek pleasure or escape discomfort, but over time, the behavior takes on a life of its own, becoming a compulsive cycle that feels impossible to break. This definition applies equally to the consumption of pornography and the act of masturbation when they cross the threshold from occasional habits to compulsions.

The brain's reward system plays a central role in addiction. This system, designed to reinforce behaviors that are beneficial for survival, is driven by dopamine—a neurotransmitter associated with pleasure, motivation, and reinforcement. When you engage in rewarding activities, such as eating or socializing, your brain releases dopamine to signal that the behavior is positive and should be repeated. However, pornography and compulsive masturbation hijack this system, providing artificially high levels of stimulation that far exceed what natural rewards can offer.

Each time you consume pornography or engage in compulsive masturbation, your brain releases a surge of dopamine. This creates a powerful sense of pleasure and reinforces the behavior, encouraging you to repeat it. Over time, the brain begins to adapt by reducing its sensitivity to dopamine—a process known as tolerance. As a result, you may find yourself seeking more frequent or intense stimulation to achieve the same level of satisfaction, leading to a cycle of escalating use.

What distinguishes addiction from mere enjoyment is the loss of control. While occasional indulgence in pleasurable activities is a normal part of life, addiction occurs when the behavior becomes compulsive—when you feel unable to stop even as it interferes with other areas of your life. For example, you might find yourself repeatedly viewing pornography despite feelings of guilt, or prioritizing masturbation over responsibilities, relationships, or personal goals. This loss of control is a hallmark of addiction and signals the need for intervention.

Another key aspect of addiction is its ability to override rational decision-making. The prefrontal cortex, the part of the brain responsible for self-control and long-term planning, often takes a backseat when addiction is in play. Instead, the brain's more primitive reward circuits dominate, prioritizing immediate gratification over the long-term consequences of the behavior. This is why people struggling with addiction often describe feeling as though they are acting against their own will or better judgment.

Compounding the problem is the emotional and psychological role that addiction plays. Many individuals turn to pornography or masturbation as a way to cope with stress, loneliness, boredom, or other negative emotions. These behaviors provide a temporary escape, offering a momentary sense of relief or comfort. However, because they do not address the root causes of these emotions, the relief is fleeting. This often leads to a cycle of using these behaviors to avoid discomfort, followed by feelings of guilt or dissatisfaction, which then drive further use.

It is also important to understand the environmental and societal factors that contribute to addiction. The digital age has made pornography more accessible than ever before, with explicit content available at the touch of a button. The anonymity of online platforms removes the social barriers that might have previously deterred consumption, while the endless variety of content provides a constant stream of novelty. This combination of accessibility, anonymity, and novelty makes pornography particularly addictive, as it caters directly to the brain's desire for immediate and varied rewards.

The consequences of addiction extend beyond the immediate behavior. Emotionally, addiction can lead to feelings of shame, isolation, and a diminished sense of self-worth. Socially, it can strain relationships, as compulsive behaviors often take precedence over genuine connection. Physically, excessive masturbation can sometimes result in fatigue or discomfort, while the time spent on these behaviors detracts from other pursuits, creating a sense of stagnation or unfulfilled potential.

Recognizing what addiction is and how it operates is the first step toward overcoming it. Addiction is not a moral failing or a sign of weakness—it is a condition rooted in the brain's wiring and shaped by environmental influences. Understanding this allows you to approach your recovery with compassion rather than judgment. It empowers you to take control of your behavior and begin building a life free from the constraints of addiction.

Recovery from addiction is a journey of self-discovery and growth. It requires a willingness to confront uncomfortable truths, to reflect on the factors that drive your behavior, and to take intentional steps toward change. While the process is not easy, it is deeply rewarding, offering the chance to reclaim your freedom, rebuild your confidence, and create a life that aligns with your values and aspirations. Addiction may be a part of your story, but it does not define you. With understanding, effort, and the right tools, you can break free from its grip and move toward a future of self-respect and fulfillment.

1.2. The Science Behind Pornography and Masturbation Addiction

The science behind pornography and masturbation addiction reveals a deeply intricate interplay between the brain's reward systems, psychological mechanisms, and the environment. Understanding these biological and neurological underpinnings is essential to recognizing why these behaviors become addictive and how they impact both the mind and body. By grasping these mechanisms, you can develop strategies to counteract their influence and work toward recovery.

At the core of pornography and masturbation addiction lies the brain's reward system, which is designed to reinforce behaviors necessary for survival and well-being. This system operates through a network of neurotransmitters, with dopamine playing a central role. Dopamine is often referred to as the "feel-good" chemical, as it creates sensations of pleasure and motivates behaviors by signaling that an activity is rewarding and worth repeating. In a natural context, dopamine is released during activities such as eating, socializing, or engaging in intimate relationships, ensuring that these behaviors are prioritized.

However, pornography and compulsive masturbation hijack this system, providing levels of stimulation that far exceed those offered by natural rewards. When viewing pornography, the brain experiences a surge of dopamine that creates a powerful sense of pleasure and excitement. The novelty and variety inherent in online pornography amplify this effect, as the brain is wired to respond strongly to new and different stimuli. Each new video, scene, or image provides a fresh burst of dopamine, keeping the viewer engaged and seeking more.

Over time, this overstimulation leads to a phenomenon known as desensitization. As the brain is exposed to repeated and intense dopamine surges, it begins to adapt by reducing the number of dopamine receptors or their sensitivity. This adaptation diminishes the brain's response to dopamine, requiring increasingly intense or novel stimuli to achieve the same level of pleasure. This explains why individuals often escalate their use of pornography, seeking more explicit or extreme content to recapture the initial high.

Compounding this issue is the strengthening of neural pathways associated with addictive behaviors. Each time a behavior is repeated, the brain reinforces the connections between the neurons involved, making it easier and more automatic to engage in that behavior in the future. This is particularly true for habitual actions like seeking out pornography or masturbating, where the repetition creates deeply ingrained patterns that are difficult to break. These patterns are often reinforced by environmental triggers—specific times, places, or emotions that are associated with the behavior—making it feel almost automatic to engage in the activity when these triggers are present.

The prefrontal cortex, the part of the brain responsible for decision-making, self-control, and long-term planning, also plays a critical role in addiction. In individuals struggling with addiction, the prefrontal cortex often becomes less effective at regulating impulses and resisting cravings. This impairment is due, in part, to the dominance of the brain's reward circuits, which prioritize immediate gratification over long-term consequences. This is why individuals often describe feeling as though they are acting against their own will, unable to stop behaviors even when they recognize their negative impact.

Pornography and masturbation addiction also interact with the brain's emotional centers, such as the amygdala, which processes emotions like stress, fear, and pleasure. For many, these behaviors serve as a coping mechanism for managing negative emotions or stressors. The temporary relief or distraction they provide reinforces the cycle, as the brain learns to associate these activities with comfort or escape. However, this relief is short-lived and does not address the underlying emotional issues, leading to repeated use and deeper entrenchment of the addictive patterns.

The digital age has significantly exacerbated the addictive potential of pornography. The ease of access, anonymity, and endless variety of content available online create an environment where compulsive use is not only possible but highly likely. The constant availability of novelty is particularly problematic, as it exploits the brain's natural preference for new stimuli, keeping users engaged far longer than they might intend. This constant stimulation can alter the brain's baseline levels of arousal and reward, making it difficult to find satisfaction in other areas of life.

The effects of pornography and masturbation addiction are not limited to the brain. Over time, these behaviors can have a cascading impact on mental, emotional, and physical health. Individuals may experience increased anxiety, depression, or feelings of isolation as a result of their addiction. Relationships can suffer due to decreased intimacy, unrealistic expectations, or a lack of emotional connection. Physically, excessive masturbation can lead to fatigue, discomfort, or even reduced sexual sensitivity, further compounding the negative effects.

Understanding the science behind pornography and masturbation addiction highlights the importance of approaching recovery with both compassion and strategy. Addiction is not a moral failing or a lack of willpower; it is a condition rooted in the brain's natural processes, amplified by environmental factors and personal circumstances. By recognizing these mechanisms, you can begin to disrupt the patterns that sustain addiction and replace them with healthier, more fulfilling behaviors.

Recovery is a process of retraining the brain, restoring balance to the reward system, and reestablishing control over your choices. This involves not only addressing the behavior itself but also understanding and managing the triggers, emotions, and thought patterns that drive it. Armed with knowledge of the science behind addiction, you are better equipped to navigate this journey and reclaim your life with confidence and self-respect.

1.3. How Addiction Develops: Triggers and Habits

Addiction to pornography and masturbation does not occur overnight. It develops gradually, shaped by patterns of behavior, psychological triggers, and environmental influences that reinforce these habits over time. Understanding how addiction develops—how triggers and habits interact to create a cycle of dependency—is essential for breaking free and regaining control over your actions. By identifying the mechanisms that sustain addiction, you can begin to dismantle them and build healthier patterns that align with your values and goals.

At the heart of addiction is a cycle that repeats itself, driven by a combination of emotional needs, external cues, and the brain's reward system. This cycle often begins with a trigger—an internal or external stimulus that prompts a desire to engage in the addictive behavior. Triggers can vary widely and may include stress, boredom, loneliness, or specific environmental cues such as being alone or having access to a device. For many, these triggers are tied to emotional states that feel uncomfortable or overwhelming, such as anxiety, frustration, or sadness.

When a trigger occurs, it activates the brain's reward circuitry, creating a craving for the pleasure or relief associated with the addictive behavior. In the case of pornography and masturbation, the craving may manifest as a strong urge to seek out explicit content or engage in the behavior as a way to escape or distract from the trigger. This craving is reinforced by the anticipation of the dopamine rush that these activities provide—a sensation that temporarily alleviates discomfort and creates a sense of gratification.

Once the behavior is engaged, it reinforces the neural pathways in the brain associated with the addiction. Each repetition strengthens these connections, making the behavior more automatic and less conscious over time. This is why addiction often feels like a reflex or compulsion, as though the behavior happens without deliberate thought. The relief or pleasure experienced during the behavior serves as a reward, solidifying the association between the trigger, the action, and the outcome.

However, the relief provided by these behaviors is short-lived. After the dopamine surge subsides, individuals often experience a crash, characterized by feelings of guilt, shame, or dissatisfaction. These negative emotions not only diminish the initial sense of relief but also create new triggers, perpetuating the cycle. For example, the guilt of engaging in the behavior may lead to stress or sadness, which then becomes a trigger for seeking comfort through the same behavior. This self-perpetuating loop is what makes addiction so difficult to break.

Habits play a significant role in sustaining addiction. A habit is a behavior that has been repeated enough times to become automatic, requiring little conscious effort or decision-making. In the context of addiction, habits are formed around the routines and rituals associated with the behavior. For instance, you may find yourself instinctively reaching for your phone or computer at specific times of the day or in response to particular emotions. These habitual patterns are reinforced by the brain's tendency to prioritize efficiency, creating shortcuts that bypass conscious thought.

Breaking the cycle of addiction requires disrupting these habits and replacing them with healthier alternatives. This begins with identifying your triggers and understanding the specific cues that prompt the behavior. By bringing awareness to these triggers, you can begin to anticipate and prepare for them, reducing their power to compel you into action. For example, if loneliness is a trigger, you might develop strategies to connect with others or engage in activities that provide emotional fulfillment without resorting to addictive behaviors.

Equally important is examining the rewards associated with the behavior and finding alternative ways to meet the underlying needs it fulfills. If stress relief is a primary driver of your addiction, you might explore relaxation techniques such as deep breathing, mindfulness, or physical exercise as substitutes. These healthier options can provide the same sense of relief without the negative consequences of addiction.

Another key aspect of breaking the cycle is understanding the role of routines in reinforcing addictive behaviors. Many addictions thrive on predictability and repetition, making it essential to disrupt the patterns that support them. This might involve changing your environment, altering your daily schedule, or introducing new habits that redirect your energy and attention. For instance, if your addiction is tied to specific times of day, you might plan activities during those times that keep you engaged and focused elsewhere.

It's also important to recognize that breaking free from addiction is a process, not a one-time event. The patterns and habits that sustain addiction are deeply ingrained, and it takes time and effort to replace them with healthier alternatives. Setbacks are a natural part of this journey and should not be viewed as failures. Instead, they provide valuable opportunities to learn about your triggers, refine your strategies, and strengthen your commitment to change.

Understanding how addiction develops—how triggers, habits, and rewards interact to create a cycle of dependency—empowers you to take intentional steps toward recovery. By identifying the patterns that sustain your addiction, you can begin to disrupt them and create new pathways that support your well-being and long-term goals. This process requires patience, persistence, and self-compassion, but it also offers the opportunity for profound growth and transformation. Each step you take toward breaking the cycle is a step closer to reclaiming your freedom and building a life that reflects your true values and aspirations.

1.4. Emotional and Psychological Effects of Addiction

The emotional and psychological effects of addiction to pornography and masturbation run deep, often affecting every aspect of a person's life. While the behavior itself might seem isolated to moments of indulgence, its consequences ripple through mental health, self-esteem, relationships, and overall well-being. Understanding these effects is critical for recognizing the broader impact of addiction and motivating the journey toward recovery.

One of the most pervasive emotional consequences of addiction is the experience of guilt and shame. Many individuals struggling with compulsive pornography use or masturbation find themselves trapped in a cycle of behavior that conflicts with their personal values or aspirations. They may feel ashamed of their inability to stop, guilty for hiding their behavior from loved ones, or embarrassed about the time and energy spent on these activities. These emotions can erode self-worth, creating a negative self-image that reinforces the cycle of addiction. Instead of motivating change, guilt and shame often lead to feelings of hopelessness, making it harder to break free.

Beyond guilt and shame, addiction frequently fosters feelings of isolation. The secretive nature of pornography use and masturbation often means that these behaviors are hidden from others, creating a sense of separation from friends, family, or partners. Over time, this secrecy can evolve into a broader emotional withdrawal, where individuals avoid social interactions or meaningful connections due to fear of judgment or rejection. This isolation not only exacerbates the emotional toll of addiction but also deprives individuals of the support systems that could help them recover.

Addiction also has a profound impact on self-esteem. The repetitive nature of compulsive behaviors can make individuals feel powerless, as though they have lost control over their actions. This perceived lack of control often leads to self-criticism and a diminished sense of self-worth. Individuals may begin to see themselves solely through the lens of their addiction, defining their identity by their struggles rather than their strengths or accomplishments. This distorted self-perception can become a barrier to recovery, as it undermines the confidence needed to pursue change.

Psychologically, addiction to pornography and masturbation can create distorted beliefs and expectations about intimacy and relationships. Pornography, in particular, often portrays unrealistic scenarios that prioritize physical gratification over emotional connection. Regular exposure to such content can alter perceptions of what intimacy should look like, leading to dissatisfaction in real-life relationships. Individuals may struggle to form meaningful connections, as their expectations are shaped by an artificial and often unattainable standard. This disconnect can result in feelings of loneliness and frustration, further perpetuating the cycle of addiction.

The emotional and psychological effects of addiction extend to the brain's reward system, which becomes desensitized over time. As the brain adapts to the repeated dopamine surges caused by pornography and masturbation, it becomes less responsive to everyday pleasures. This desensitization can lead to a condition known as anhedonia, where individuals find it difficult to experience joy or satisfaction in activities that once brought them happiness. This diminished capacity for pleasure contributes to feelings of emptiness or dissatisfaction, further driving addictive behaviors as individuals seek to recapture the sense of reward.

Addiction also impacts emotional regulation, making it harder to cope with stress, anxiety, or other negative emotions. Many individuals turn to pornography or masturbation as a way to escape or numb difficult feelings, creating a dependency on these behaviors as a form of emotional self-medication. However, this reliance on addiction as a coping mechanism prevents individuals from developing healthier strategies for managing their emotions. Over time, this can result in a reduced ability to navigate life's challenges, leading to increased vulnerability to stress and emotional instability.

Another significant psychological effect of addiction is the erosion of trust, both in oneself and in relationships with others. For individuals in committed partnerships, addiction can create feelings of betrayal or inadequacy in their partners, leading to tension and conflict. The secrecy surrounding the behavior often compounds these issues, as partners may feel excluded or deceived. On a personal level, addiction can undermine self-trust, as individuals repeatedly make promises to stop only to find themselves unable to follow through. This erosion of trust can create a sense of disconnection, both internally and externally.

The cumulative effect of these emotional and psychological consequences is a profound sense of disempowerment. Addiction takes a toll on an individual's ability to live in alignment with their values, pursue their goals, and engage fully in their relationships and personal growth. It narrows the focus of life to the addictive behavior, diminishing opportunities for fulfillment and leaving individuals feeling stuck or stagnant.

Recognizing these effects is an essential step in the recovery process. By understanding how addiction impacts your emotions, thoughts, and behaviors, you can begin to see the broader context of your struggle. This awareness not only highlights the need for change but also provides motivation to pursue it. The emotional and psychological toll of addiction is not insurmountable. With the right tools and support, it is possible to rebuild self-esteem, repair relationships, and rediscover joy and purpose in life.

Recovery is not just about stopping a behavior; it is about reclaiming your sense of self and restoring balance to your mental and emotional well-being. It requires addressing the root causes of addiction, developing healthier ways to manage emotions, and rebuilding trust in yourself and others. Each step you take toward understanding and overcoming these effects is a step closer to living a life free from the constraints of addiction, filled with self-respect, connection, and fulfillment.

1.5. The Impact on Relationships and Daily Life

The impact of addiction to pornography and masturbation extends far beyond the individual. It can infiltrate relationships and daily life, creating a ripple effect of challenges that strain personal connections, disrupt routines, and undermine emotional well-being. Understanding these impacts is crucial not only for recognizing the broader consequences of addiction but also for finding the motivation to work toward recovery and restore balance in your life.

One of the most immediate and visible impacts of addiction is on personal relationships. Intimacy, both physical and emotional, forms the foundation of meaningful connections, yet addiction often creates barriers to fostering this closeness. Pornography, in particular, can distort perceptions of intimacy by prioritizing physical gratification over emotional connection. Over time, individuals may find it difficult to engage fully with their partners, as their expectations and desires are shaped by the unrealistic scenarios portrayed in explicit content. This disconnect can lead to feelings of dissatisfaction, frustration, or inadequacy on both sides of the relationship.

For partners of individuals struggling with addiction, the effects can be deeply personal and painful. Many partners report feeling excluded, betrayed, or unimportant, particularly when the addictive behavior is hidden or secretive. They may question their own worth or desirability, interpreting their partner's addiction as a reflection of their inadequacy. This can lead to tension, misunderstandings, and conflict, straining the trust and mutual respect that form the foundation of a healthy relationship. In some cases, the emotional distance created by addiction can result in the breakdown of the relationship altogether.

Beyond romantic relationships, addiction can also affect connections with friends, family, and colleagues. The time and energy devoted to compulsive behaviors often come at the expense of social interactions and meaningful engagements. Individuals may withdraw from others, either out of shame about their behavior or simply because their addiction consumes the time they would otherwise spend nurturing relationships. Over time, this isolation can lead to feelings of loneliness and disconnection, further fueling the addictive cycle as individuals turn to these behaviors for comfort or escape.

The impact of addiction on daily life is equally significant. Time, one of the most valuable resources, is often squandered in pursuit of the addictive behavior. Hours spent seeking out and engaging in pornography or masturbation can interfere with responsibilities, personal goals, and self-care. This diversion of time and energy can lead to a sense of stagnation, as individuals find themselves unable to make progress in areas that matter most to them, such as their careers, education, or personal development.

Addiction can also disrupt routines and create a lack of structure in daily life. Many individuals find that their addictive behaviors become intertwined with specific times, places, or activities, creating patterns that are difficult to break. For example, someone might develop a habit of watching pornography late at night, leading to sleep deprivation and decreased productivity the following day. These disruptions can accumulate over time, impacting not only the individual but also those who rely on them, such as family members or coworkers.

Emotionally, addiction often creates a sense of internal conflict and dissatisfaction. Individuals may feel torn between their desire to stop and their inability to control their behavior, leading to frustration and self-criticism. This internal struggle can manifest as anxiety, irritability, or a lack of focus, making it harder to engage fully in daily activities or enjoy life's simple pleasures. Over time, the emotional toll of addiction can contribute to more serious mental health challenges, such as depression or chronic stress.

The financial impact of addiction is another consideration. While pornography is often free, some individuals may find themselves spending money on subscriptions, pay-per-view content, or other related expenses. These costs, while seemingly small in isolation, can add up over time and create financial strain, particularly when compounded by the loss of productivity or career setbacks caused by the addiction. The guilt and stress associated with financial mismanagement can further exacerbate the emotional toll of addiction.

Addiction also affects physical well-being. Excessive masturbation, for instance, can lead to fatigue, physical discomfort, or reduced sexual sensitivity, while the sedentary nature of these behaviors can contribute to a decline in overall health. Over time, these physical effects can create a cycle of inactivity and neglect, where individuals prioritize their addiction over exercise, nutrition, or other forms of self-care.

Perhaps one of the most insidious impacts of addiction is its ability to erode a sense of purpose and fulfillment. When addiction takes hold, it narrows the focus of life to the behavior itself, crowding out opportunities for growth, connection, and personal achievement. Individuals may find themselves stuck in a loop of short-term gratification, unable to pursue the long-term goals and aspirations that bring meaning to life. This sense of stagnation can be deeply demoralizing, reinforcing the cycle of addiction and making it harder to break free.

Recognizing the impact of addiction on relationships and daily life is an important step in the recovery process. It allows you to see the broader context of your behavior, not as a source of guilt or shame but as a motivation for change. By understanding how addiction affects those around you and your ability to live a balanced, fulfilling life, you can begin to identify the areas where recovery will have the greatest impact.

Breaking free from addiction is not just about stopping a behavior —it's about reclaiming your time, energy, and potential. It's about rebuilding trust, fostering meaningful connections, and creating a life that reflects your values and aspirations. The challenges may be significant, but so are the rewards: a renewed sense of purpose, deeper relationships, and the freedom to live fully and authentically. Each step you take toward recovery is a step toward restoring the balance and harmony that addiction has disrupted, both in your own life and in the lives of those around you.

1.6. Myths and Misconceptions About Porn and Masturbation

The topic of pornography and masturbation is often surrounded by myths and misconceptions that can distort our understanding of addiction and its effects. These false beliefs can create unnecessary shame, minimize the seriousness of the issue, or lead individuals to underestimate the challenges of recovery. Disentangling these myths from the facts is essential for developing a clear and compassionate perspective on addiction, as well as for fostering the mindset needed to overcome it.

One of the most pervasive myths is that pornography and masturbation are harmless activities with no long-term consequences. While it is true that occasional indulgence in these behaviors does not automatically lead to addiction, repeated and compulsive use can have profound effects on mental health, relationships, and overall well-being. Addiction to pornography and masturbation often develops gradually, making it easy to dismiss or overlook its impact until it becomes deeply entrenched. This misconception can prevent individuals from recognizing the problem early and taking steps to address it.

Another common misconception is that addiction to pornography or masturbation is simply a matter of weak willpower or poor self-control. This belief stigmatizes those who struggle with addiction, framing their behavior as a personal failing rather than a complex interplay of biological, psychological, and environmental factors. Addiction is not a reflection of moral weakness; it is a condition rooted in the brain's reward system, shaped by patterns of behavior, and reinforced by triggers and habits. Viewing it as such allows for a more compassionate and effective approach to recovery.

There is also a widespread belief that addiction to pornography or masturbation affects only certain types of people. Some assume that this issue is limited to those who lack discipline, face relationship difficulties, or lead lonely lives. In reality, addiction can affect anyone, regardless of their age, gender, background, or circumstances. The accessibility and anonymity of online pornography make it particularly easy for individuals from all walks of life to develop problematic habits. Recognizing the universal nature of this issue helps to reduce stigma and opens the door for more open conversations and understanding.

A particularly harmful myth is the idea that quitting pornography or masturbation is easy or that individuals can stop simply by deciding to do so. While some people may be able to change their habits with relative ease, many find that breaking free from addiction requires significant effort, self-reflection, and support. The neural pathways reinforced by addictive behaviors do not disappear overnight, and recovery often involves a gradual process of rewiring the brain and replacing old habits with healthier ones. Dismissing the challenges of recovery can lead to frustration and self-blame when progress is slower than expected.

Another misconception is that all use of pornography or masturbation is inherently harmful or indicative of addiction. It is important to differentiate between occasional, consensual, and intentional engagement in these behaviors and compulsive use that interferes with daily life and well-being. Not everyone who consumes pornography or masturbates is addicted, and not all instances of these behaviors have negative consequences. Addiction is characterized by loss of control, escalation, and negative impact, and understanding these distinctions is key to addressing the issue appropriately.

Some believe that addiction to pornography or masturbation is a purely personal issue that does not affect others. This myth overlooks the ways in which addiction can ripple out to impact relationships, work, and family life. Partners may feel neglected or betrayed, friendships may suffer due to withdrawal or secrecy, and professional responsibilities may be compromised by a lack of focus or time management. Recognizing the broader impact of addiction underscores the importance of addressing it, not only for the individual but also for their loved ones and communities.

The myth that shame and guilt are necessary for recovery is another barrier to progress. While it is natural to feel regret or disappointment about the effects of addiction, excessive shame often backfires, deepening the cycle of dependency. Shame can make individuals feel unworthy of change or incapable of overcoming their struggles, creating a sense of hopelessness that undermines recovery efforts. A more constructive approach is to cultivate self-compassion, acknowledging the challenges of addiction while committing to the work of healing and growth.

A related misconception is the belief that professional help is the only effective solution for addiction. While therapy and support groups can be invaluable for many, self-therapy is also a viable and empowering path to recovery. By equipping individuals with tools for self-awareness, emotional regulation, and habit change, self-therapy allows them to take charge of their recovery in a way that is accessible and flexible. Understanding that there are multiple routes to healing can help individuals find the approach that works best for them.

Lastly, there is the myth that recovery means eliminating all desire or thoughts related to sexuality. Recovery is not about suppressing natural human instincts but about restoring balance and control. The goal is to develop a healthy relationship with sexuality, one that aligns with your values and supports your well-being. By addressing the underlying causes of addiction and learning healthier ways to manage desires and emotions, it is possible to embrace sexuality as a positive and fulfilling part of life.

Dispelling these myths and misconceptions is a critical step in overcoming addiction to pornography and masturbation. It creates a clearer understanding of the challenges involved and fosters a more compassionate perspective on the journey to recovery. By replacing false beliefs with accurate information, you can approach your struggle with greater confidence and self-respect, knowing that change is possible and that you are not alone. Recovery is a process that requires effort, patience, and support, but it is also a path to freedom, growth, and a renewed sense of self.

Chapter 2:
Recognizing the Signs

Recognizing the signs of addiction is a crucial step toward recovery. Often, the behaviors associated with addiction to pornography and masturbation become so ingrained in daily life that they are difficult to distinguish from routine habits or coping mechanisms. This chapter is designed to help you develop a deeper awareness of your patterns, triggers, and emotional responses, so you can identify when these behaviors have crossed the line into addiction.

Understanding the signs of compulsive behavior is about more than labeling or diagnosing yourself—it's about gaining clarity and insight into how these patterns are affecting your life. Addiction is often accompanied by emotional, behavioral, and relational red flags that signal the need for change. These signs can manifest in subtle ways, such as a growing sense of dissatisfaction, or in more obvious disruptions to your daily routines, relationships, and responsibilities.

Awareness is the foundation of change. By identifying the specific ways in which addiction shows up in your life, you can begin to understand its impact and take intentional steps to address it. This process involves honest self-reflection, a willingness to confront uncomfortable truths, and a commitment to observing your behavior without judgment. The goal is not to punish yourself for the past but to equip yourself with the knowledge and tools to create a healthier future.

This chapter will guide you through the process of recognizing the signs of addiction, from identifying compulsive behaviors to understanding the emotional and psychological cues that sustain them. You will learn how to assess your triggers, recognize the role of shame and guilt in the cycle of addiction, and track your progress toward recovery. By bringing these patterns into focus, you can take the first steps toward breaking free from their grip and reclaiming control over your choices.

Recognizing the signs is not just about acknowledging the presence of addiction; it's about empowering yourself to make informed and intentional changes. As you move through this chapter, remember that self-awareness is not about perfection but about progress. Each insight you gain brings you closer to understanding your behaviors and, ultimately, to breaking free from their constraints. Recovery begins with recognition, and this chapter provides the roadmap for that essential first step.

2.1. Identifying Compulsive Behaviors

Identifying compulsive behaviors is the first step toward understanding and addressing addiction. Compulsion, by its nature, involves an overwhelming urge to perform a behavior repeatedly, even when it interferes with your well-being or conflicts with your values. In the context of pornography and masturbation addiction, compulsive behaviors often manifest as habits that feel out of your control, driven by triggers, and reinforced by short-term relief or pleasure. Recognizing these patterns is essential for regaining control and beginning the journey toward recovery.

One of the defining characteristics of compulsive behavior is a sense of urgency or inevitability. You may feel a strong, almost irresistible pull to engage in the behavior, even if part of you wishes to resist. This internal conflict—knowing that the behavior is not serving your best interests but feeling powerless to stop—can be a clear indicator of compulsion. This is particularly true when the behavior is performed automatically or habitually, without conscious decision-making.

Compulsive behaviors are often accompanied by an inability to moderate or stop, despite efforts to do so. You might set intentions or make promises to yourself to reduce or eliminate the behavior, only to find yourself slipping back into old patterns. This repeated cycle of trying and failing can create feelings of frustration, guilt, or shame, further entrenching the compulsion. Over time, this loss of control becomes a hallmark of addiction, signaling the need for intervention.

Another key aspect of compulsive behavior is its impact on your life. When pornography and masturbation begin to consume excessive amounts of time or interfere with your responsibilities, relationships, or personal goals, they have crossed the line from occasional indulgence to problematic patterns. You might notice that you are procrastinating on work, neglecting social interactions, or sacrificing sleep to engage in these behaviors. These disruptions can accumulate, leading to a sense of stagnation or disconnection from the things that matter most.

Triggers play a significant role in driving compulsive behaviors. Triggers can be external, such as being alone, using certain devices, or encountering specific media, or internal, such as feelings of stress, boredom, or loneliness. Recognizing your triggers is a vital part of identifying compulsive patterns. For example, you might notice that you are more likely to engage in the behavior during moments of emotional vulnerability or when you are in particular environments. Understanding these cues allows you to anticipate and address them, reducing their power over your actions.

Compulsive behaviors often follow a predictable pattern or cycle. This cycle typically begins with a trigger, followed by a craving or urge to engage in the behavior. Once the behavior is performed, it provides temporary relief or pleasure, reinforcing the pattern. However, this relief is often short-lived and followed by negative emotions such as guilt, shame, or dissatisfaction. These emotions then act as new triggers, perpetuating the cycle. Breaking this cycle requires not only recognizing the behavior but also understanding the mechanisms that sustain it.

An important clue in identifying compulsive behavior is the presence of escalation. Over time, you may find that the behaviors that once provided satisfaction no longer have the same effect. This can lead to seeking more frequent or intense engagement, such as consuming more explicit or novel content or increasing the frequency of masturbation. Escalation is a sign that the brain's reward system has become desensitized, requiring greater stimulation to achieve the same level of pleasure. This pattern of escalation is a key marker of addiction.

Emotional cues also offer valuable insights into compulsive behavior. You might notice that certain feelings consistently precede or follow the behavior, such as anxiety, loneliness, frustration, or sadness. These emotional patterns provide clues about the role the behavior plays in your life—whether as a coping mechanism, a distraction, or a source of comfort. By identifying these emotional connections, you can begin to explore alternative ways to address your needs and manage your emotions.

Another sign of compulsive behavior is the secrecy or concealment that often accompanies it. You may go to great lengths to hide your actions from others, feeling embarrassed or ashamed about what you are doing. This secrecy can create a sense of isolation, as it prevents you from seeking support or sharing your struggles with trusted friends or loved ones. The need to hide the behavior is often a sign that it is causing internal conflict and interfering with your sense of integrity.

Finally, compulsive behaviors are often accompanied by a sense of dissatisfaction or lack of fulfillment. Even as you engage in the behavior, you may feel that it is not providing the gratification or meaning you hoped for. This disconnect between expectation and reality can create a cycle of chasing fleeting rewards, leaving you feeling empty or unfulfilled. Recognizing this dissatisfaction is an important step in understanding the broader impact of the behavior and finding motivation to pursue change.

Identifying compulsive behaviors is not about judgment or self-criticism; it is about bringing awareness to the patterns that are shaping your life. By observing your actions, triggers, and emotional responses with honesty and curiosity, you can begin to understand the role that pornography and masturbation play in your life. This awareness lays the foundation for breaking free from these patterns and building a healthier relationship with yourself and your choices. Recovery starts with recognition, and each insight you gain is a step toward reclaiming control and creating a life of purpose and fulfillment.

2.2. When Masturbation Becomes a Problem

Recognizing when masturbation becomes a problem is a critical step in understanding the line between healthy behavior and addiction. Masturbation, like any natural and normal human behavior, can exist on a spectrum. For many, it is a healthy way to explore sexuality, relieve stress, or satisfy curiosity. However, when it crosses certain boundaries, it can lead to significant emotional, psychological, and relational challenges. Identifying these boundaries requires self-awareness, honesty, and a willingness to confront the patterns in your life that may no longer serve you.

Masturbation becomes problematic when it transitions from an occasional or intentional act into a compulsive behavior that feels uncontrollable. This loss of control is a hallmark of addiction, characterized by an inability to stop or reduce the behavior despite efforts to do so. You might find yourself making promises to limit or eliminate masturbation, only to repeat the behavior shortly after. This cycle of trying and failing can lead to frustration, self-doubt, and feelings of helplessness, further reinforcing the compulsion.

One of the clearest indicators that masturbation has become a problem is its frequency. While there is no universally "normal" number of times for masturbation, engaging in it excessively—particularly to the point where it interferes with your daily life—can be a sign of an underlying issue. If masturbation is consuming a significant amount of your time, causing you to neglect responsibilities, or interfering with your ability to maintain healthy routines, it may have crossed into problematic territory.

Another key sign is the emotional impact of the behavior. Masturbation should not leave you feeling guilty, ashamed, or disconnected. If these negative emotions consistently follow the act, it could indicate that the behavior is at odds with your values, goals, or sense of self. Over time, these emotions can erode your self-esteem, creating a cycle of guilt and shame that perpetuates the compulsion. This emotional toll is often compounded by the secrecy that surrounds problematic behaviors, as individuals may feel the need to hide their actions from others, further isolating themselves.

Masturbation can also become problematic when it is used as a primary coping mechanism for stress, loneliness, or other emotional challenges. While occasional use of masturbation to manage emotions is not inherently harmful, relying on it as a habitual escape can prevent you from developing healthier ways to address your feelings. Over time, this dependency can hinder emotional growth and resilience, making it harder to navigate life's challenges without resorting to the behavior.

Another red flag is when masturbation begins to replace or negatively affect real-life relationships. If you find yourself choosing masturbation over meaningful interactions with others, or if your ability to connect with partners is diminished due to the frequency or nature of the behavior, it may be time to reassess its role in your life. This is particularly true if the behavior is accompanied by pornography use, which can distort perceptions of intimacy and create unrealistic expectations that strain relationships.

Physical effects can also signal that masturbation has become problematic. Excessive masturbation can lead to fatigue, discomfort, or reduced sensitivity, which may interfere with your sexual health and overall well-being. These physical consequences, while often reversible, are a sign that your body is being pushed beyond its limits. Listening to your body and recognizing when it is signaling distress is an important part of maintaining a healthy balance.

The presence of escalation is another indicator that masturbation has crossed into problematic territory. Escalation occurs when the behavior becomes increasingly frequent, intense, or extreme over time. You may find that what once satisfied you no longer has the same effect, leading you to seek out more frequent or varied stimulation. This pattern of escalation is a common feature of addiction, as the brain adapts to repeated dopamine surges and requires greater stimulation to achieve the same level of pleasure.

Masturbation can also become problematic when it creates a sense of dependency. If you feel unable to relax, focus, or sleep without engaging in the behavior, it may be playing an outsized role in your life. Dependency often arises when masturbation is tied to specific routines, environments, or emotional states, creating a cycle that feels difficult to break. This sense of reliance can undermine your autonomy and make it harder to develop alternative strategies for meeting your needs.

The impact of problematic masturbation often extends to other areas of life, such as work, education, or hobbies. If the behavior is causing you to procrastinate, miss deadlines, or underperform in areas that are important to you, it is a sign that it is interfering with your ability to live a balanced and fulfilling life. Similarly, if you find that you are prioritizing masturbation over activities that once brought you joy or satisfaction, it may be time to examine its role in your daily routine.

Recognizing when masturbation becomes a problem is not about labeling the behavior as inherently good or bad. Instead, it is about understanding its impact on your life and assessing whether it aligns with your values, goals, and overall well-being. By observing the frequency, emotional effects, and consequences of the behavior with honesty and curiosity, you can gain clarity about its role in your life and decide whether it is time to make a change.

This awareness is the first step toward breaking free from problematic patterns and reclaiming control over your choices. Masturbation, like any behavior, should serve your well-being rather than detract from it. By addressing the underlying triggers, emotions, and routines that sustain compulsive patterns, you can develop a healthier relationship with yourself and your desires, paving the way for a more balanced and fulfilling life. Recovery is not about eliminating a behavior entirely; it is about restoring balance, intention, and self-respect.

2.3. Emotional and Behavioral Red Flags

Recognizing emotional and behavioral red flags is an essential part of understanding when addiction to pornography and masturbation is taking a toll on your mental health and daily life. These red flags are often subtle at first, but as they accumulate, they can disrupt your emotional well-being, relationships, and overall sense of self. Identifying these signs is not about assigning blame or shame but about cultivating awareness and taking steps to address the patterns that no longer serve you.

One of the most common emotional red flags is the presence of guilt and shame. After engaging in the behavior, you may feel an overwhelming sense of regret, disappointment, or even self-loathing. These feelings often stem from the internal conflict between your actions and your values or goals. While guilt can sometimes serve as a motivator for change, excessive shame often becomes a barrier, creating a cycle where negative emotions drive further engagement in the behavior as a means of escape. This loop of guilt, shame, and compulsion can be challenging to break without recognizing its role in sustaining the addiction.

Another emotional indicator is a growing sense of dissatisfaction or emptiness. The temporary relief or pleasure provided by pornography and masturbation may no longer feel as fulfilling as it once did, leaving you with a lingering sense of unease or frustration. This disconnect between the anticipated reward and the actual experience often signals that the behavior is no longer serving a healthy purpose. Over time, this dissatisfaction can contribute to feelings of apathy, reduced motivation, and a lack of engagement in other areas of life.

Behaviorally, one of the clearest red flags is the inability to stop or moderate the behavior despite repeated efforts. You may find yourself setting boundaries or making promises to limit your engagement, only to revert to old patterns. This loss of control is a defining feature of addiction and can create a sense of powerlessness or frustration. The more frequently this cycle repeats, the stronger the compulsion becomes, making it harder to break free without intentional intervention.

Escalation is another key behavioral sign. Over time, you may find that the frequency, intensity, or nature of your behaviors increases. For example, you might spend more time seeking out pornography, explore more extreme or novel content, or engage in masturbation more frequently to achieve the same level of satisfaction. This escalation often reflects the brain's adaptation to repeated dopamine surges, which reduces sensitivity to the reward and drives the need for greater stimulation.

Isolation is a significant red flag, both emotionally and behaviorally. You may begin to withdraw from social interactions, avoiding friends, family, or partners due to feelings of shame or fear of judgment. This withdrawal often extends to activities you once enjoyed, as the addictive behavior consumes more of your time and energy. Over time, isolation can deepen feelings of loneliness and disconnection, further fueling the cycle of addiction as you seek comfort or distraction through the behavior.

Another behavioral indicator is the neglect of responsibilities and priorities. You may notice that your engagement in pornography or masturbation interferes with your ability to meet work deadlines, study effectively, or fulfill commitments to others. Procrastination, decreased productivity, and a lack of focus often accompany addiction, as the behavior takes precedence over other aspects of life. This neglect can lead to a sense of stagnation or unfulfilled potential, further compounding emotional distress.

Secrecy and deception are also common behavioral red flags. You may find yourself hiding your actions from others, feeling the need to cover up your behaviors or lie about how you spend your time. This secrecy often creates a sense of internal conflict, as it undermines trust in your relationships and your own sense of integrity. The effort required to maintain this façade can be emotionally exhausting and isolating, reinforcing feelings of shame and disconnection.

Emotionally, addiction often manifests as heightened irritability or mood swings. The reliance on pornography and masturbation as a coping mechanism for stress or negative emotions can reduce your ability to manage these feelings effectively in other areas of life. As a result, you may find yourself becoming more reactive, impatient, or easily frustrated. These emotional shifts can strain relationships and create additional stress, perpetuating the cycle of addiction.

Over time, these emotional and behavioral patterns can lead to a diminished sense of self-worth. You may begin to view yourself through the lens of your addiction, focusing on your perceived failures rather than your strengths or achievements. This negative self-perception can create a feedback loop, where feelings of inadequacy or hopelessness drive further engagement in the behavior as a form of escape. Breaking free from this loop requires recognizing that addiction does not define you and that change is both possible and within your reach.

Recognizing emotional and behavioral red flags is not about self-judgment but about cultivating self-awareness. By observing these patterns with honesty and compassion, you can begin to understand how addiction is affecting your life and take steps to address it. Each red flag offers an opportunity to reflect, learn, and grow, providing the foundation for meaningful and lasting change.

The journey to recovery begins with awareness. By identifying the signs that pornography and masturbation are interfering with your emotional and behavioral well-being, you can take the first steps toward breaking free from their grip. This process requires patience, perseverance, and a commitment to self-compassion, but it also offers the opportunity to rebuild your sense of self-worth, restore balance in your life, and rediscover the joy and fulfillment that addiction may have taken away.

2.4. Assessing Your Triggers

Understanding and assessing your triggers is a pivotal step in breaking free from addiction to pornography and masturbation. Triggers are the catalysts—internal or external cues—that initiate the cycle of addictive behavior. They act as signals to the brain, prompting cravings and the compulsion to engage in the behavior. Recognizing and addressing these triggers can help you regain control and develop healthier responses to the challenges they present.

Triggers can be broadly categorized into two types: external and internal. External triggers are situational or environmental factors that create an urge to engage in the addictive behavior. These might include being alone, having access to a smartphone or computer, seeing suggestive images, or being in specific locations where the behavior commonly occurs. Internal triggers, on the other hand, are emotional or psychological states, such as stress, boredom, loneliness, anxiety, or even feelings of excitement or accomplishment. Both types of triggers play a role in reinforcing the cycle of addiction, and both require mindful attention to break the patterns they create.

Assessing your triggers begins with cultivating self-awareness. This involves observing your behaviors and emotions without judgment, identifying patterns in when, where, and why you feel compelled to engage in pornography or masturbation. For example, you might notice that the urge arises more frequently during moments of stress or when you are feeling lonely. By tracking these occurrences, you can begin to understand the specific situations or feelings that act as triggers for you.

A helpful tool in this process is keeping a trigger journal. In this journal, you can record details about each time you feel an urge to engage in the behavior. Note the time, location, emotional state, and any external factors that might have contributed to the urge. Over time, patterns will emerge, revealing the most common and powerful triggers in your life. This increased awareness allows you to anticipate and prepare for these situations, reducing their power to control your actions.

One of the challenges of addressing triggers is that they often operate subconsciously. For instance, you might find yourself reaching for your phone or opening a browser without consciously deciding to do so. These automatic behaviors are the result of deeply ingrained neural pathways formed through repetition. To disrupt these pathways, it is essential to bring your triggers into conscious awareness, pausing to reflect on what is driving the behavior before acting on it.

Another important aspect of assessing triggers is understanding the emotional needs they represent. Triggers often point to underlying feelings or unmet needs that the addictive behavior is attempting to address. For example, if stress is a common trigger for you, it may indicate a need for relaxation or relief from pressure. If loneliness is a trigger, it might point to a desire for connection or intimacy. By identifying these needs, you can begin to explore healthier ways to fulfill them, such as practicing mindfulness for stress relief or reaching out to friends and loved ones for support.

In some cases, triggers may be tied to specific routines or habits. For example, you might have developed a pattern of engaging in the behavior at a particular time of day, such as before bed or during a break from work. These habitual triggers can be particularly challenging because they are reinforced by repetition and familiarity. Addressing them requires disrupting the routines that support them and replacing them with new, healthier habits. For instance, you might establish a new bedtime routine that includes reading, journaling, or meditation, creating a positive and intentional way to end your day.

It's also important to recognize the role of technology in creating and reinforcing triggers. The constant availability of devices and the internet makes it easy for external triggers to arise, often without warning. Notifications, advertisements, or even idle browsing can unexpectedly lead to urges. Setting boundaries around technology use—such as implementing content filters, turning off notifications, or designating device-free times and spaces—can help reduce the influence of these triggers.

Dealing with triggers also involves building emotional resilience. Internal triggers, such as stress or boredom, often stem from an inability to manage certain feelings effectively. Developing skills to cope with these emotions can weaken their ability to prompt addictive behavior. Practices such as mindfulness, deep breathing, exercise, or creative hobbies can provide healthy outlets for stress and boredom, reducing the need to turn to pornography or masturbation as a coping mechanism.

While it's impossible to eliminate all triggers from your life, you can learn to respond to them in healthier and more intentional ways. This process involves creating a pause between the trigger and the behavior, giving yourself time to reflect and choose a different course of action. For example, if a trigger arises, you might take a moment to step away, engage in a grounding activity, or remind yourself of your goals and motivations for change.

Understanding your triggers is not about avoiding responsibility or blaming external factors; it's about gaining clarity and taking proactive steps to address the influences that drive your behavior. By assessing your triggers with honesty and curiosity, you can begin to break the automatic cycle of addiction and regain control over your choices. Each trigger you identify and address is an opportunity to grow stronger in your recovery and closer to the life you want to create.

Recovery is not about eliminating every challenge or temptation from your life but about learning to navigate them with confidence and resilience. By recognizing your triggers and developing strategies to manage them, you can build the skills needed to break free from the grip of addiction and move toward a healthier, more intentional way of living. This process takes time and patience, but each step you take brings you closer to a future of freedom and self-respect.

2.5. The Role of Shame and Guilt in Addiction

Shame and guilt are powerful emotions that often play a central role in the cycle of addiction to pornography and masturbation. These feelings can act as both triggers and consequences, creating a feedback loop that reinforces the very behavior they are tied to. Understanding the role of shame and guilt in addiction is essential for breaking this cycle and building a healthier relationship with yourself.

Guilt typically arises when you perceive that your actions have violated your own moral or personal standards. It is a natural emotional response to behavior that conflicts with your values or expectations of yourself. For many individuals struggling with addiction, guilt becomes a frequent companion, surfacing after each instance of engaging in the behavior. While guilt can sometimes motivate change, excessive or unresolved guilt often backfires, creating feelings of hopelessness or inadequacy that make recovery even more challenging.

Shame, on the other hand, is a more pervasive and internalized emotion. Unlike guilt, which focuses on a specific action ("I did something wrong"), shame attacks your sense of self ("I am wrong"). Shame convinces you that your behavior defines your worth, painting you as unworthy, unlovable, or irredeemable. This self-judgment can be crippling, undermining your confidence and making it difficult to believe in your ability to change.

In the context of addiction, shame and guilt often work together to create a vicious cycle. After engaging in the addictive behavior, you may feel an immediate sense of guilt for violating your values or commitments. This guilt can quickly spiral into shame, as you begin to internalize negative beliefs about yourself, such as "I'm weak" or "I'm a failure." These feelings of inadequacy and self-loathing can then serve as triggers, driving you to seek temporary relief or escape through the very behavior you are trying to overcome.

Compounding this cycle is the secrecy that often surrounds addiction. Many individuals struggling with pornography and masturbation feel compelled to hide their behavior from others, fearing judgment or rejection. This secrecy reinforces feelings of shame and isolation, creating additional barriers to seeking help or support. Over time, the silence surrounding the behavior can make it feel even more overwhelming, as though it is an insurmountable burden that must be carried alone.

It is important to recognize that shame and guilt, while painful, are not inherently bad or wrong. They are emotional signals, pointing to areas where your actions are out of alignment with your values or desires. However, when these emotions become chronic or overwhelming, they can hinder rather than help your recovery. The key is to address shame and guilt in a way that fosters growth and healing, rather than allowing them to perpetuate the cycle of addiction.

One of the most effective ways to break free from shame and guilt is to practice self-compassion. Self-compassion involves treating yourself with the same kindness, understanding, and support that you would offer to a close friend or loved one. It means acknowledging your struggles without judgment, recognizing that addiction is a challenge rather than a personal failing. By cultivating self-compassion, you create a space where you can learn from your experiences and take steps toward change without being paralyzed by self-criticism.

Reframing your perspective on guilt can also be helpful. Instead of viewing guilt as a sign of failure, see it as a reminder of your values and a motivator for aligning your actions with those values. Guilt can serve as a guide, helping you identify the areas where you want to grow and make changes. When approached with curiosity rather than condemnation, guilt can be a constructive force in your recovery journey.

Shame, however, often requires a more intentional effort to dismantle. Because shame attacks your sense of self-worth, it is important to challenge the beliefs and narratives that sustain it. This might involve reminding yourself that addiction is not a reflection of your character but a condition rooted in brain chemistry, habits, and environmental factors. It might also involve seeking out supportive relationships or communities where you can share your struggles without fear of judgment, fostering a sense of connection and understanding.

Another way to address shame and guilt is to focus on small, achievable steps toward change. Each positive action you take, no matter how small, reinforces your belief in your ability to grow and improve. Over time, these steps build momentum, helping you break free from the cycle of negative emotions and addictive behaviors. Celebrate your progress, and remember that recovery is not about perfection but about persistence and resilience.

It is also essential to recognize when shame and guilt are becoming overwhelming and to seek help if needed. Speaking with a trusted friend, counselor, or support group can provide relief and perspective, helping you process your emotions in a healthy way. External support can remind you that you are not alone and that your struggles do not define your worth.

Understanding the role of shame and guilt in addiction is not about eliminating these emotions entirely but about learning to navigate them with compassion and self-awareness. By addressing these feelings constructively, you can begin to break the cycle of addiction and build a healthier, more positive relationship with yourself. Recovery is not just about changing your behavior; it is about reclaiming your sense of self-worth and creating a life that reflects your values, aspirations, and inherent dignity.

2.6. How to Measure Your Progress

Measuring your progress is a vital part of overcoming addiction to pornography and masturbation. Recovery is a journey, and tracking your growth allows you to recognize how far you've come, identify areas that need more attention, and stay motivated along the way. Addiction can often create a distorted sense of failure or stagnation, especially when setbacks occur, so having tangible measures of progress is essential to maintaining focus and confidence. This process is not about perfection but about celebrating the small wins that accumulate into significant change.

One of the first steps in measuring your progress is to establish a clear baseline. This involves taking an honest look at your current behaviors, triggers, and patterns. Reflect on questions like how often you engage in the addictive behavior, what emotional or situational triggers are involved, and how the addiction impacts your daily life. This baseline provides a starting point from which you can measure growth and identify trends over time. While this process can feel uncomfortable, it is a necessary step in understanding where you are and what you want to change.

Setting realistic and specific goals is another critical component of tracking progress. Recovery goals should be measurable and actionable, such as reducing the frequency of the behavior, developing healthier coping mechanisms, or building new habits that support your overall well-being. For example, you might aim to go a certain number of days without engaging in the behavior or to replace one instance of compulsion with a positive activity, such as exercise or meditation. These goals give you a framework for evaluating your efforts and recognizing improvements.

Journaling can be a powerful tool for measuring progress. Keeping a record of your thoughts, feelings, and behaviors allows you to identify patterns and reflect on your journey. In your journal, you can track the frequency and intensity of urges, the strategies you use to resist them, and your emotional responses before and after each challenge. Over time, your entries will provide valuable insights into your triggers, coping mechanisms, and overall trajectory. They will also serve as a reminder of the progress you've made, even when it feels slow or difficult.

Another way to measure progress is to evaluate your ability to manage triggers and emotional responses. As you become more aware of your triggers and develop healthier coping strategies, you will likely notice a decrease in the frequency or intensity of cravings. For instance, a trigger that once felt overwhelming may become more manageable as you learn to pause, reflect, and choose a different response. Recognizing these shifts, no matter how small, is an important indicator of growth.

Changes in your daily life and routines are also valuable markers of progress. Addiction often disrupts sleep, productivity, relationships, and self-care, so improvements in these areas can signal recovery. You might notice that you're sleeping better, focusing more effectively at work, spending more time with loved ones, or engaging in hobbies that bring you joy. These changes reflect a shift in priorities and a growing ability to create a life that aligns with your values and aspirations.

Emotional resilience is another important measure of progress. Recovery is not just about eliminating a behavior but about building the emotional skills needed to navigate life's challenges. Pay attention to how you handle stress, boredom, or negative emotions as you progress. Are you finding it easier to sit with discomfort without resorting to the addictive behavior? Are you able to recognize and address your feelings with greater clarity and self-compassion? These are signs that you are developing the tools needed for lasting change.

It's also helpful to periodically reflect on your overall sense of self-worth and confidence. Addiction often erodes self-esteem, leaving individuals feeling powerless or unworthy. As you progress, you may notice a renewed sense of pride in your ability to make intentional choices and overcome challenges. This growing confidence reinforces your belief in your capacity for change and serves as a foundation for continued growth.

While it's important to measure progress, it's equally crucial to approach this process with flexibility and self-compassion. Recovery is rarely a straight line, and setbacks are a natural part of the journey. Rather than viewing setbacks as failures, see them as opportunities to learn and refine your approach. Each challenge you face provides valuable insights into your triggers, coping mechanisms, and areas that need more attention. By treating yourself with kindness and understanding, you create a supportive environment for growth.

Celebrate your victories, no matter how small they may seem. Each day without engaging in the addictive behavior, each instance of resisting a trigger, and each moment of self-awareness is a step forward. Acknowledge these achievements and use them as motivation to keep going. Recovery is a collection of small, consistent steps, and recognizing these moments of progress builds momentum and reinforces your commitment to change.

Finally, consider seeking feedback from trusted friends, family members, or support groups. External perspectives can provide valuable insights into how your behavior and mindset are evolving. They can also offer encouragement, accountability, and a sense of connection, reminding you that you are not alone in your journey.

Measuring your progress is about more than tracking numbers or milestones—it's about cultivating self-awareness, celebrating growth, and maintaining motivation. Recovery is a dynamic and ongoing process, and each step you take brings you closer to reclaiming your life and creating a future of freedom, balance, and fulfillment. By recognizing and appreciating your progress, you can stay focused on your goals and continue moving forward with confidence and self-respect.

Chapter 3:
Building a Foundation for Change

Building a strong foundation for change is the cornerstone of recovery from addiction to pornography and masturbation. Without a solid base, attempts to change can feel fleeting or unsustainable, leaving you frustrated and uncertain about the path forward. This chapter is designed to guide you in laying the groundwork for meaningful and lasting transformation, emphasizing the importance of self-awareness, realistic goals, discipline, and emotional resilience.

Recovery is not just about stopping a behavior—it is about creating a life that reflects your values, aspirations, and sense of purpose. This requires looking beyond the surface of your actions to understand the deeper patterns, triggers, and emotional needs that drive them. By cultivating self-awareness, you can begin to identify these underlying factors and take intentional steps to address them. Awareness is the first step toward reclaiming control and creating change that feels authentic and empowering.

Setting realistic goals is another essential part of building a foundation for recovery. Change rarely happens all at once; it is a gradual process that involves consistent effort and incremental progress. By breaking your journey into manageable steps, you can stay focused, motivated, and less overwhelmed. These goals serve as markers of progress and give you a clear sense of direction, helping you stay on track even when challenges arise.

Understanding the role of discipline and willpower is also critical. Recovery often requires you to make difficult choices, resisting the pull of familiar patterns in favor of healthier alternatives. While willpower alone is not enough to overcome addiction, it is an important tool in navigating moments of temptation and building new habits. This chapter will explore how to cultivate discipline in a way that feels sustainable and supportive, rather than rigid or punitive.

Creating a supportive environment is equally important. The spaces we inhabit and the people we surround ourselves with can either hinder or help our efforts to change. By intentionally shaping your environment to reduce triggers and promote positive behaviors, you can set yourself up for success. This might involve physical changes, such as limiting access to certain devices, or relational changes, such as seeking out people who uplift and encourage you.

Finally, emotional self-care is a fundamental component of recovery. Addiction often serves as a coping mechanism for managing difficult emotions, so learning to address these feelings in healthy ways is key to breaking the cycle. This chapter will guide you in developing practices that nurture your emotional well-being, such as mindfulness, self-compassion, and stress management. By prioritizing your emotional health, you can create a foundation for growth that supports all aspects of your recovery.

Building a foundation for change is not about achieving perfection; it is about creating a strong and stable base from which you can grow. Each step you take toward understanding yourself, setting goals, and creating a supportive environment brings you closer to reclaiming your life. This chapter will provide you with the tools and insights needed to begin this process, empowering you to take control and build a future of freedom, purpose, and fulfillment.

3.1. The Power of Self-Awareness

The power of self-awareness lies at the heart of recovery from addiction to pornography and masturbation. Self-awareness is the ability to observe and understand your thoughts, emotions, and behaviors without judgment, allowing you to identify the patterns that sustain addiction and the triggers that perpetuate the cycle. It is the first step toward taking control of your actions and building a healthier, more intentional life. Without self-awareness, change is difficult, as the mechanisms driving your behavior remain hidden and unchallenged.

Developing self-awareness begins with a willingness to look inward, even when what you see may be uncomfortable. Addiction often thrives in the shadows of denial, secrecy, or avoidance. By bringing your behaviors into the light of awareness, you disrupt the automatic nature of addiction and open the door to intentional action. This process is not about blaming yourself or dwelling on mistakes but about cultivating curiosity and understanding. It's about asking questions like, "Why do I feel compelled to engage in this behavior?" or "What emotions or situations trigger my urges?"

One of the most effective tools for building self-awareness is mindfulness. Mindfulness involves paying attention to your present moment experience with openness and acceptance. When applied to recovery, mindfulness helps you observe your urges, thoughts, and feelings as they arise, without immediately acting on them. For example, instead of automatically reaching for your phone or seeking out pornography when you feel stressed, you might take a moment to pause, notice the sensation of stress in your body, and acknowledge the urge without judgment. This simple act of observation creates space between the trigger and the behavior, giving you the opportunity to choose a different response.

Journaling is another powerful practice for cultivating self-awareness. Writing down your thoughts, feelings, and experiences allows you to track patterns and identify the underlying factors driving your behavior. You can use your journal to reflect on questions such as: What was I feeling when the urge arose? What triggered the urge? How did I respond, and what was the outcome? Over time, this practice can reveal valuable insights into the emotional and situational contexts of your addiction, empowering you to address them more effectively.

Self-awareness also involves recognizing your triggers—both internal and external. Internal triggers may include emotions like stress, loneliness, boredom, or frustration, while external triggers might involve specific times of day, locations, or access to certain devices. By identifying these triggers, you can begin to anticipate and prepare for them, reducing their power to compel you into automatic behavior. For example, if you notice that you often feel the urge to engage in the behavior when you are alone at night, you might plan alternative activities during that time, such as reading, meditating, or connecting with a friend.

Another key aspect of self-awareness is understanding the emotional needs that your addiction may be masking. Addiction often serves as a coping mechanism for unmet needs, such as the need for connection, relaxation, or distraction. By exploring these underlying needs, you can begin to develop healthier ways to meet them. For instance, if you realize that your addiction is driven by a desire for connection, you might focus on strengthening your relationships or finding new ways to connect with others. If it stems from a need for relaxation, you might explore practices like yoga, deep breathing, or creative hobbies.

Self-awareness also involves acknowledging the impact of your behavior on your life and the lives of those around you. This includes recognizing how addiction affects your mental health, relationships, productivity, and overall well-being. While this awareness can be painful, it is also a powerful motivator for change. It allows you to see the broader context of your actions and understand the stakes of your recovery. This understanding can inspire a deeper commitment to breaking free from addiction and creating a life aligned with your values.

As you cultivate self-awareness, it's important to approach yourself with compassion rather than criticism. Addiction is not a reflection of your worth or character; it is a condition shaped by complex factors, including brain chemistry, habits, and environmental influences. Treating yourself with kindness and understanding creates a supportive foundation for growth. Instead of focusing on what you perceive as failures, celebrate your willingness to learn, reflect, and take steps toward change.

The journey of self-awareness is ongoing, as new insights and challenges arise throughout the recovery process. Each moment of self-discovery brings you closer to understanding yourself and your behavior, empowering you to make intentional choices that align with your goals. By developing this awareness, you are not only addressing the patterns of addiction but also building a stronger connection with yourself—a connection rooted in honesty, curiosity, and self-respect.

Ultimately, self-awareness is about reclaiming your power. It allows you to move from a place of reactivity to one of intentionality, where your actions are guided by your values and aspirations rather than by automatic impulses. This shift is transformative, enabling you to break free from the constraints of addiction and create a life of freedom, purpose, and fulfillment. Each step you take in cultivating self-awareness is a step toward reclaiming your life and embracing the person you want to become.

3.2. Setting Realistic Goals for Recovery

Setting realistic goals for recovery is a cornerstone of the journey to overcoming addiction to pornography and masturbation. Goals serve as a roadmap, guiding your efforts and providing a sense of direction and purpose. However, to be effective, they must be realistic, achievable, and tailored to your individual circumstances. Unrealistic or overly ambitious goals can lead to frustration, disappointment, and a sense of failure, while well-crafted goals can inspire confidence, build momentum, and sustain your motivation.

The first step in setting realistic goals is to acknowledge where you are in your recovery journey. Honesty with yourself about your current habits, triggers, and challenges is essential. Recovery is not a one-size-fits-all process, and your goals should reflect your unique experiences and needs. Whether you are just beginning to explore the idea of change or have already made strides in reducing the behavior, your goals should align with your starting point and provide a manageable path forward.

Breaking larger goals into smaller, actionable steps is a key strategy for making them realistic. For example, if your ultimate goal is to eliminate compulsive behavior entirely, start by focusing on achievable milestones, such as reducing the frequency of the behavior over time. Instead of aiming to stop immediately and completely, you might set a goal to go one day, then three days, and eventually a week without engaging in the behavior. These incremental steps allow you to build confidence and experience success, which can motivate you to continue progressing.

Another important aspect of realistic goal-setting is ensuring that your goals are specific and measurable. Vague goals like "stop watching pornography" or "improve my habits" lack clarity and make it difficult to track progress. Instead, frame your goals in concrete terms, such as "reduce pornography use to once a week within the next month" or "replace nightly masturbation with a relaxation routine three times this week." Specific goals give you a clear target to aim for and a way to evaluate your efforts.

It's also crucial to set goals that are time-bound but flexible. Recovery is a process, and rigid timelines can create unnecessary pressure or feelings of failure if progress is slower than expected. While it's helpful to establish timeframes for your goals, be open to adjusting them as needed based on your experiences. For example, if you set a goal to avoid pornography for 30 days but find it challenging to reach that milestone, extend the timeline or break it into smaller intervals. The focus should be on progress, not perfection.

Balancing short-term and long-term goals is another key consideration. Short-term goals provide immediate focus and a sense of accomplishment, while long-term goals represent the broader vision for your recovery. For instance, a short-term goal might be to go one day without engaging in the behavior, while a long-term goal could involve building a life where your actions align with your values and priorities. Both types of goals work together, with short-term successes contributing to long-term achievements.

Self-reflection is an important part of setting and revising your goals. Take time to consider what motivates you and what outcomes you hope to achieve through recovery. Are you seeking to improve your relationships, enhance your mental health, or gain more time and energy for meaningful pursuits? Understanding your "why" gives your goals deeper significance and helps you stay committed even when challenges arise. Revisit your motivations regularly to remind yourself of the purpose behind your efforts.

While setting goals, it's also important to anticipate obstacles and plan for how you will navigate them. Triggers, stress, and setbacks are natural parts of the recovery process, and preparing for them can make them less disruptive. For example, if you know that boredom is a trigger, include a goal to develop new hobbies or activities to fill your time. If stress often leads to compulsive behavior, set a goal to practice stress management techniques, such as mindfulness or exercise. Proactively addressing potential challenges ensures that your goals remain realistic and achievable.

Celebrate your successes, no matter how small they may seem. Recovery is a journey of incremental progress, and each step forward is a victory worth acknowledging. Celebrating milestones reinforces your belief in your ability to change and provides positive reinforcement for your efforts. Whether it's a day, a week, or a month of progress, take time to recognize your achievements and the hard work they represent.

Finally, approach goal-setting with self-compassion. Recovery is not a linear process, and setbacks are a natural part of the journey. If you don't achieve a goal as quickly or fully as you hoped, avoid self-criticism and focus on what you can learn from the experience. Adjust your goals as needed and remind yourself that growth takes time. The key is to remain committed to the process and to view each step, even the challenging ones, as part of your overall progress.

Setting realistic goals is about creating a framework that supports your growth and keeps you moving forward. By breaking down your aspirations into manageable steps, grounding them in self-awareness, and remaining flexible and compassionate, you can build momentum and confidence in your ability to overcome addiction. Each goal you set and achieve brings you closer to reclaiming your life and creating a future that reflects your values, freedom, and fulfillment.

3.3. Understanding the Role of Discipline and Willpower

Understanding the role of discipline and willpower in recovery from addiction to pornography and masturbation is vital to creating sustainable change. While neither discipline nor willpower alone can fully address the complexities of addiction, they are essential tools in navigating the challenges of breaking old habits and building new, healthier patterns. Recovery requires a combination of intentional effort, self-reflection, and emotional growth, with discipline and willpower serving as foundational elements of this process.

Discipline, at its core, is the ability to make consistent choices aligned with your goals and values, even in the face of temptation or discomfort. It is about creating structure and routine in your life that supports your recovery and reduces the likelihood of falling back into old patterns. Discipline is not about perfection or rigidity; it is about persistence and the willingness to prioritize long-term growth over short-term gratification.

Willpower, on the other hand, is the capacity to resist urges and impulses in the moment. It is the mental energy that allows you to pause, reflect, and choose a course of action that aligns with your recovery goals. While willpower is an important resource, it is not infinite. Like a muscle, it can become fatigued with overuse, which is why relying solely on willpower to overcome addiction is rarely effective. Instead, willpower should be used strategically, alongside other tools and strategies that support your journey.

One of the first steps in cultivating discipline is to establish a clear vision of your goals and values. Reflect on what you hope to achieve through recovery and why these goals are meaningful to you. This deeper sense of purpose will serve as a guiding force when challenges arise, helping you stay committed even when the path feels difficult. Write down your goals and values, and revisit them regularly to reinforce your motivation.

Creating a structured daily routine is another powerful way to build discipline. Addiction often thrives in unstructured or idle moments, where triggers and urges have more room to take hold. By filling your day with purposeful activities, you reduce opportunities for compulsive behavior and create a sense of momentum and accomplishment. Your routine might include practices like exercise, meditation, journaling, or pursuing hobbies that bring you joy and fulfillment. These activities not only occupy your time but also reinforce your commitment to living in alignment with your values.

Discipline also involves anticipating and addressing triggers. Knowing what situations, emotions, or environments tend to lead to compulsive behavior allows you to prepare and respond proactively. For example, if you know that boredom often triggers your urges, you can plan engaging activities to fill your free time. If certain times of day are particularly challenging, you can schedule constructive tasks or set reminders to stay focused on your goals. By reducing the influence of triggers, you create an environment that supports your recovery.

Willpower comes into play during moments of temptation, where you must make a conscious choice to resist the urge and redirect your energy. Strengthening willpower requires practice and intentionality. One effective technique is the "pause and reflect" method. When you feel an urge arise, take a moment to pause, breathe deeply, and reflect on your goals and values. Remind yourself of the reasons you are working toward recovery and the positive outcomes you want to achieve. This pause creates space between the trigger and the response, giving you the opportunity to choose a healthier course of action.

Another way to strengthen willpower is to build small, achievable habits that reinforce your commitment to change. For example, you might set a goal to spend five minutes each day practicing mindfulness or to replace one instance of compulsive behavior with a positive activity. These small wins build confidence and reinforce your ability to make intentional choices, creating a foundation for larger changes over time.

It's important to recognize that both discipline and willpower are finite resources that can be depleted by stress, fatigue, or emotional challenges. This is why self-care and emotional regulation are critical components of recovery. Ensuring that you get enough sleep, eat well, and manage stress effectively helps replenish your mental energy and strengthens your ability to stay disciplined. Similarly, developing healthy ways to cope with emotions, such as journaling, talking to a friend, or practicing relaxation techniques, reduces the likelihood of turning to addictive behaviors for relief.

Another aspect of discipline is learning to forgive yourself when setbacks occur. Recovery is not a linear process, and moments of struggle are inevitable. Instead of viewing these moments as failures, see them as opportunities to learn and grow. Reflect on what led to the setback, and use that insight to refine your strategies and strengthen your resolve. Self-compassion is a vital part of discipline, as it allows you to move forward with a renewed sense of purpose rather than becoming stuck in self-criticism.

Accountability can also play a significant role in reinforcing discipline and willpower. Sharing your goals with a trusted friend, partner, or support group creates a sense of responsibility and encouragement. Knowing that others are aware of your journey can motivate you to stay committed and provide valuable feedback and support when challenges arise. Surrounding yourself with people who uplift and inspire you strengthens your ability to persevere.

Ultimately, discipline and willpower are tools that empower you to take control of your choices and create a life aligned with your aspirations. While they require effort and practice, they also offer the freedom and fulfillment that come with living intentionally. By combining these tools with self-awareness, emotional growth, and a supportive environment, you can navigate the challenges of recovery and move closer to the life you envision for yourself. Each moment of discipline and willpower is a step toward reclaiming your life and building a future of purpose and self-respect.

3.4. Creating a Supportive Environment

Creating a supportive environment is a critical component of recovery from addiction to pornography and masturbation. The spaces you inhabit and the people you surround yourself with can either reinforce unhealthy patterns or provide a foundation for positive change. By intentionally shaping your environment to minimize triggers and foster growth, you set yourself up for success in your recovery journey. This process involves not only making physical and practical changes but also cultivating relationships and habits that align with your goals.

The first step in creating a supportive environment is to identify the elements of your surroundings that contribute to addictive behaviors. These might include access to devices, certain times of day when you're alone, or locations where the behavior has become habitual. Recognizing these patterns allows you to take proactive steps to reduce their influence. For example, if late-night access to your phone or computer is a common trigger, consider implementing boundaries such as keeping devices out of your bedroom or setting a specific time to turn off screens each night.

Technology, in particular, plays a significant role in reinforcing addiction to pornography. The internet offers instant access to explicit content, often with minimal barriers. To counteract this, consider using tools and settings that help limit exposure to triggers. Content filters, website blockers, and accountability software can be effective in reducing temptation and creating a sense of structure around your online activities. While these tools are not a cure-all, they can provide a helpful buffer, allowing you to focus on building healthier habits.

Another important aspect of creating a supportive environment is rethinking your routines and habits. Addiction often thrives in unstructured or idle moments, so establishing a daily routine that prioritizes meaningful activities can help fill your time with purpose. This might involve setting specific times for exercise, work, hobbies, or social interactions, creating a framework that supports your recovery. For example, if evenings are a particularly vulnerable time, you might schedule a relaxing activity like reading, meditation, or journaling to replace the behavior.

Physical changes to your environment can also make a significant difference. Rearranging your living space to reflect your recovery goals can serve as a powerful reminder of your commitment to change. This might involve creating a designated space for mindfulness practices, removing items associated with addictive behaviors, or organizing your surroundings to promote a sense of calm and focus. Even small changes, such as adding inspiring quotes or personal affirmations to your workspace, can reinforce your motivation.

The social aspect of your environment is equally important. The people you interact with can have a profound impact on your recovery, either supporting or hindering your progress. Surrounding yourself with individuals who uplift, encourage, and hold you accountable can make the journey feel less isolating. Share your goals with trusted friends or family members who can offer understanding and support. Consider joining a recovery group or community, where you can connect with others who are navigating similar challenges. These connections provide not only emotional support but also valuable insights and strategies for overcoming addiction.

In some cases, creating a supportive environment may involve distancing yourself from relationships or situations that trigger or reinforce addictive behaviors. This can be a difficult but necessary step, especially if certain individuals or dynamics contribute to feelings of stress, shame, or temptation. Setting boundaries with people who do not respect your recovery goals is an act of self-care that prioritizes your well-being.

It's also important to cultivate an internal environment of self-compassion and resilience. The way you speak to yourself and handle setbacks plays a significant role in your ability to recover. Practice reframing negative self-talk into constructive and encouraging language. For instance, instead of saying, "I'm a failure for giving in to my urges," you might say, "I faced a challenge, and I can learn from this experience to make better choices next time." This internal support creates a mental environment that fosters growth and persistence.

Part of creating a supportive environment is recognizing and celebrating your progress. Recovery is a journey of incremental steps, and acknowledging your achievements—no matter how small— reinforces your commitment to change. This could involve tracking your milestones in a journal, rewarding yourself for reaching specific goals, or simply taking a moment to reflect on how far you've come. These acts of recognition provide motivation and affirm your ability to succeed.

Finally, remember that creating a supportive environment is an ongoing process. As you progress in your recovery, new challenges and triggers may arise, requiring adjustments to your surroundings and strategies. Stay attuned to what works for you and be willing to adapt. Recovery is not about creating a perfect environment but about fostering one that continually supports your growth and resilience.

By intentionally shaping your physical, social, and mental environment, you create the conditions for meaningful and lasting change. Each adjustment you make, no matter how small, is a step toward reclaiming control and building a life that aligns with your values and aspirations. A supportive environment is not just a tool for recovery—it is a reflection of your commitment to yourself and your future.

3.5. The Importance of Emotional Self-Care

Emotional self-care is a cornerstone of recovery from addiction to pornography and masturbation. Often, these behaviors develop as a response to unresolved emotional needs or as a way to cope with stress, loneliness, boredom, or other difficult feelings. By prioritizing emotional self-care, you can address these underlying drivers and build a foundation of resilience, self-awareness, and well-being. This process involves learning to identify and honor your emotions, developing healthy coping strategies, and fostering a deeper connection with yourself.

At its core, emotional self-care begins with self-awareness. Addiction often thrives in an environment of avoidance, where uncomfortable emotions are suppressed or ignored rather than acknowledged and processed. Developing the ability to recognize and name your emotions is the first step in breaking this cycle. When you feel the urge to engage in the behavior, pause and ask yourself what you are feeling in that moment. Are you stressed, anxious, lonely, or frustrated? Identifying these emotions helps you understand the role they play in driving your behavior and opens the door to healthier ways of addressing them.

Once you've identified your emotions, it's important to validate them without judgment. Many people struggling with addiction experience shame or guilt about their feelings, seeing them as weaknesses or flaws. However, emotions are a natural and integral part of the human experience, and acknowledging them with compassion is essential for emotional self-care. Remind yourself that it's okay to feel whatever you're feeling and that your emotions are valid, even if they are challenging or uncomfortable.

Healthy coping strategies are a key component of emotional self-care. Addiction often serves as a maladaptive way of managing emotions, providing temporary relief or distraction but leaving the underlying issues unresolved. Developing alternative strategies allows you to address your emotional needs in ways that promote healing and growth. For example, if stress is a common trigger, practices like mindfulness, deep breathing, or yoga can help you find calm and balance. If loneliness is a driving factor, reaching out to a friend, joining a social group, or engaging in community activities can provide connection and support.

One of the most effective tools for emotional self-care is mindfulness. This practice involves cultivating a nonjudgmental awareness of your present-moment experience, including your thoughts, emotions, and physical sensations. Mindfulness allows you to observe your feelings without being overwhelmed by them, creating space for intentional responses rather than automatic reactions. For instance, when you notice an urge to engage in the behavior, mindfulness can help you pause, recognize the underlying emotion, and choose a healthier way to address it.

Journaling is another powerful method for processing emotions and gaining insight into your inner world. Writing about your thoughts and feelings provides an outlet for self-expression and helps you identify patterns or triggers that contribute to your addiction. Journaling can also serve as a space to reflect on your progress, celebrate your successes, and explore your goals and aspirations. Over time, this practice can deepen your understanding of yourself and strengthen your emotional resilience.

Self-compassion is a vital element of emotional self-care, particularly during the recovery process. Addiction is often accompanied by harsh self-criticism and feelings of inadequacy, which can undermine your confidence and motivation. Practicing self-compassion means treating yourself with the same kindness and understanding you would offer to a close friend. When you encounter setbacks or difficult emotions, remind yourself that recovery is a journey and that growth often involves challenges. Instead of focusing on what you perceive as failures, celebrate your efforts and progress.

Boundaries are another important aspect of emotional self-care. Protecting your emotional well-being sometimes means setting limits with others or with yourself. For example, you might need to distance yourself from people or environments that trigger negative emotions or temptations. Setting boundaries also involves saying no to commitments or activities that overwhelm you, giving yourself the space to focus on your recovery and personal growth.

Engaging in activities that bring you joy and fulfillment is a powerful way to nurture your emotional health. Addiction often narrows your focus, leaving little room for hobbies, creativity, or exploration. Reconnecting with activities you enjoy—or discovering new ones—can help you rediscover a sense of purpose and passion. Whether it's painting, gardening, playing music, or learning a new skill, these pursuits provide a positive outlet for your energy and emotions.

Physical self-care is closely tied to emotional well-being and should not be overlooked. Regular exercise, a balanced diet, and sufficient sleep all contribute to emotional stability and resilience. Physical activity, in particular, has been shown to reduce stress, improve mood, and boost self-esteem, making it an invaluable tool in the recovery process. By taking care of your body, you create a strong foundation for emotional health.

Connecting with others is another crucial element of emotional self-care. Addiction often fosters isolation, but meaningful relationships provide support, encouragement, and perspective. Sharing your journey with trusted friends, family members, or a recovery group can help you feel less alone and more understood. These connections remind you that you are not defined by your addiction and that you are deserving of love and support.

Ultimately, emotional self-care is about creating a compassionate and nurturing relationship with yourself. It is an ongoing practice of recognizing your needs, honoring your feelings, and taking intentional steps to support your well-being. By prioritizing emotional self-care, you address the underlying drivers of addiction and build the resilience needed to navigate life's challenges. Each act of self-care is a step toward reclaiming your sense of self and creating a life that reflects your values, aspirations, and inherent worth.

3.6. Finding Motivation to Break Free

Finding motivation to break free from addiction to pornography and masturbation is a deeply personal journey that requires understanding your inner drivers, connecting with your values, and building a vision of the life you want to create. Motivation is the fuel that propels you forward, even in the face of challenges, setbacks, and temptations. While it may waver at times, nurturing and sustaining your motivation is essential for making lasting change and reclaiming control over your actions and choices.

At the heart of motivation lies your "why." This is the deeper reason you want to overcome addiction and create a healthier, more fulfilling life. Your "why" might be rooted in a desire to improve your relationships, restore your self-respect, regain control of your time and energy, or align your actions with your values. Take time to reflect on what matters most to you and how breaking free from addiction supports those priorities. Writing down your reasons for recovery can provide clarity and serve as a powerful reminder when your motivation wanes.

Another way to strengthen your motivation is to visualize the life you want to create. Imagine a future where you are free from the constraints of addiction, where your time, energy, and focus are directed toward meaningful pursuits. Picture the relationships you want to nurture, the goals you want to achieve, and the sense of self-respect you want to cultivate. This vision of your future can inspire you to stay committed, even when the process feels difficult or overwhelming.

Breaking your journey into small, achievable steps can also boost motivation. Large, long-term goals can feel daunting, but focusing on immediate, manageable actions creates a sense of momentum and accomplishment. For example, instead of focusing solely on quitting entirely, set a goal to go one day without engaging in the behavior or to replace one instance of compulsion with a positive activity. Each small success builds confidence and reinforces your belief in your ability to change.

Celebrating your progress, no matter how small, is another effective way to sustain motivation. Recovery is a journey of incremental growth, and acknowledging your achievements along the way helps you stay focused and optimistic. Whether it's reaching a milestone, resisting a trigger, or simply reflecting on how far you've come, take time to recognize and appreciate your efforts. These moments of celebration remind you that progress is possible and that each step forward brings you closer to your goals.

Connecting with your values is a powerful motivator for change. Addiction often creates a sense of disconnection from your true self, as your actions may conflict with your ideals or aspirations. Reconnecting with your values—such as integrity, self-respect, or compassion—helps you realign your choices with what matters most to you. Reflect on how overcoming addiction allows you to live in greater alignment with these values, and use them as a guiding compass when faced with difficult decisions.

Understanding the costs of addiction can also serve as a motivator. Reflect on how addiction has impacted your life, including its effects on your relationships, mental health, productivity, and overall well-being. While this reflection can be uncomfortable, it provides valuable insight into why change is necessary. By recognizing the ways in which addiction has held you back, you can channel those feelings into a commitment to move forward and reclaim your life.

Building a support system is another key element of maintaining motivation. Recovery is not a journey you have to take alone, and connecting with others who understand and support your goals can provide encouragement and accountability. Whether it's a trusted friend, family member, or recovery group, sharing your experiences and progress with others can help you stay motivated and feel less isolated. Support systems also provide perspective during moments of doubt, reminding you of your strengths and resilience.

Engaging in activities that bring you joy and fulfillment is another way to foster motivation. Addiction often narrows your focus, leaving little room for hobbies, creativity, or exploration. Rediscovering what makes you happy—whether it's painting, hiking, playing music, or learning a new skill—can reignite your passion for life and remind you of the rewards of recovery. These activities also serve as positive alternatives to addictive behaviors, helping you build a life that feels rich and purposeful.

Anticipating challenges and preparing for them is an important part of staying motivated. Recovery is rarely a linear process, and setbacks are a natural part of the journey. Instead of viewing these moments as failures, see them as opportunities to learn and grow. Reflect on what led to the setback, and use that insight to refine your strategies and strengthen your resolve. Remind yourself that progress is not about perfection but about persistence and resilience.

Finally, practice self-compassion throughout your recovery journey. Motivation often falters when you are overly critical of yourself or focus on what you perceive as shortcomings. Treat yourself with the same kindness and understanding you would offer to a friend, and remind yourself that change is a process that takes time and effort. Celebrate your courage to confront addiction and your willingness to work toward a better future.

Motivation is not a fixed state but a dynamic force that ebbs and flows. By connecting with your "why," celebrating your progress, and building a vision of the life you want to create, you can sustain your commitment to recovery even during challenging times. Each step you take, no matter how small, is a testament to your strength and determination. With patience, perseverance, and self-compassion, you can break free from addiction and build a life of freedom, purpose, and fulfillment.

Chapter 4: Practical Strategies for Recovery

Practical strategies form the backbone of any successful recovery journey. While understanding the root causes of addiction and fostering self-awareness are critical first steps, translating that understanding into actionable techniques is where true transformation begins. This chapter is dedicated to equipping you with the tools and methods needed to break free from the patterns of addiction to pornography and masturbation. These strategies are designed not only to help you disrupt the cycle of addictive behavior but also to replace it with habits and routines that promote growth, resilience, and fulfillment.

The path to recovery is not about relying solely on willpower or expecting immediate change. It requires a combination of intentional actions, thoughtful planning, and consistent effort. Practical strategies provide the structure and guidance needed to navigate the challenges of recovery, offering concrete steps to address triggers, manage urges, and develop healthier alternatives. They are the building blocks of a new way of living, where your choices align with your values and aspirations.

This chapter will explore a range of approaches, from breaking the habit loop that sustains addiction to finding positive behaviors that fulfill the same needs in healthier ways. You will learn how to navigate moments of temptation, handle setbacks, and build the skills necessary to manage your emotions and responses effectively. These strategies are not one-size-fits-all; they are tools that you can adapt to your unique circumstances, ensuring they resonate with your life and goals.

One of the key aspects of practical recovery strategies is their emphasis on action. Understanding addiction is important, but taking steps to address it is what creates change. This chapter encourages you to move beyond reflection and into implementation, empowering you to reclaim control over your actions and choices. Each strategy is designed to be actionable and achievable, allowing you to build momentum and confidence as you progress.

As you explore these strategies, remember that recovery is a process of trial and learning. Some techniques may work better for you than others, and that's okay. The goal is not perfection but progress—finding what resonates with you and refining your approach as you gain experience and insight. Recovery is not about eliminating all challenges but about developing the tools and mindset to navigate them with resilience and determination.

This chapter invites you to take a proactive and empowered approach to your recovery. By embracing practical strategies, you can begin to break free from the constraints of addiction and build a life of purpose, balance, and self-respect. Each tool you use, each habit you form, and each step you take brings you closer to the freedom and fulfillment you deserve. Let these strategies guide you toward a future where your actions reflect your values, and your choices are driven by intention rather than compulsion.

4.1. Breaking the Habit Loop: Tools and Techniques

Breaking the habit loop is a critical step in overcoming addiction to pornography and masturbation. Addiction often thrives on deeply ingrained patterns that develop over time, where triggers lead to urges, and urges lead to actions. These repetitive behaviors create a loop that reinforces itself, making it difficult to break free. Understanding how this loop operates and implementing strategies to disrupt it can help you regain control and set the foundation for lasting change.

The habit loop consists of three main components: the trigger, the routine, and the reward. A trigger is any stimulus—internal or external—that initiates the cycle. This might include emotions such as stress or boredom, or environmental factors like being alone or having access to devices. The routine is the behavior itself, such as seeking out pornography or masturbating. Finally, the reward is the sense of relief, pleasure, or escape that the behavior provides. Over time, this cycle becomes automatic, as the brain associates the trigger with the behavior and the reward.

To break the habit loop, the first step is identifying your triggers. Pay close attention to the circumstances and emotions that precede your urges. Are you feeling stressed after a long day? Bored during downtime? Lonely late at night? Understanding these triggers is essential for disrupting the cycle. Keeping a journal can help you track patterns and gain clarity about the specific situations or feelings that lead to the behavior.

Once you've identified your triggers, the next step is to create a plan for managing or avoiding them. For example, if boredom is a common trigger, you might fill your schedule with engaging activities or hobbies that occupy your time and mind. If stress is a trigger, consider incorporating relaxation techniques such as deep breathing, mindfulness, or exercise into your daily routine. By addressing the triggers head-on, you reduce their power to drive the behavior.

The routine, or the behavior itself, is the second element to address. Disrupting the routine requires introducing alternative actions that provide similar rewards but align with your recovery goals. For instance, if the behavior provides relief from stress, replacing it with a healthier coping mechanism like a brisk walk or a quick journaling session can satisfy the same emotional need without reinforcing the addictive pattern. Experiment with different alternatives to find what works best for you, and make these new routines as accessible as possible to encourage their adoption.

The final component of the habit loop is the reward, which is the brain's reinforcement for engaging in the behavior. In many cases, the reward is tied to the release of dopamine, the brain's "feel-good" chemical. While the reward from addictive behaviors may be immediate and intense, it is often short-lived and followed by feelings of guilt or dissatisfaction. Recognizing this fleeting nature can help you question whether the reward is truly worth the long-term consequences.

To counteract the lure of the reward, focus on cultivating more sustainable and fulfilling sources of satisfaction. This might include pursuing creative projects, strengthening relationships, or engaging in activities that promote physical and mental well-being. Over time, as you experience the deeper rewards of these positive actions, the appeal of the addictive behavior will diminish.

Another effective strategy for breaking the habit loop is to introduce a pause between the trigger and the routine. When you feel an urge arise, take a moment to pause and reflect. Ask yourself: "What am I feeling right now? What do I need? What are my options?" This pause disrupts the automatic nature of the cycle and gives you the opportunity to make a conscious choice. Even a brief pause can create enough space to redirect your attention and energy toward a healthier alternative.

Accountability is also a powerful tool in breaking the habit loop. Sharing your goals with a trusted friend, partner, or support group creates a sense of responsibility and provides encouragement during moments of difficulty. Knowing that others are invested in your success can strengthen your resolve and remind you of the importance of your recovery. Additionally, having someone to talk to during moments of temptation can provide immediate support and perspective.

Creating a supportive environment is another key element in disrupting the habit loop. This involves removing or minimizing access to triggers and creating a space that fosters positive habits. For example, consider implementing content blockers on devices, establishing device-free zones, or setting specific times for engaging in healthy activities. These changes reduce the likelihood of encountering triggers and reinforce your commitment to change.

Breaking the habit loop also requires patience and persistence. Habits that have developed over months or years will not disappear overnight, and setbacks are a natural part of the process. Instead of viewing these moments as failures, see them as opportunities to learn and grow. Reflect on what led to the setback, and use that insight to strengthen your strategies moving forward. Each attempt to disrupt the cycle, even if imperfect, is a step toward breaking free.

Ultimately, breaking the habit loop is about reclaiming control over your choices and actions. It is a process of identifying the patterns that no longer serve you, challenging them, and replacing them with healthier alternatives. Each time you disrupt the cycle, you weaken its hold and move closer to a life of freedom, purpose, and self-respect. With consistent effort and a commitment to growth, you can overcome the patterns of addiction and build a future that reflects your values and aspirations.

4.2. Replacing Negative Behaviors with Positive Ones

Replacing negative behaviors with positive ones is a powerful strategy in overcoming addiction to pornography and masturbation. At its core, addiction often stems from unmet needs, emotional discomfort, or the desire to escape stress or boredom. While the behavior itself provides temporary relief or satisfaction, it comes at the cost of reinforcing unhealthy patterns and leaving the underlying issues unaddressed. By identifying and introducing positive alternatives, you can not only break the cycle of addiction but also build habits that enhance your well-being and align with your goals and values.

The first step in this process is to understand the specific role that the addictive behavior plays in your life. Addiction is not random; it serves a purpose, even if it's ultimately harmful. Does it help you cope with stress? Does it fill moments of boredom or loneliness? Does it provide a sense of control or escape? By identifying the emotional or psychological needs the behavior is attempting to fulfill, you can begin to explore healthier ways to address those needs.

Once you've identified the purpose of the behavior, the next step is to brainstorm positive alternatives that serve the same function but align with your recovery goals. For example, if stress is a major trigger, you might explore relaxation techniques such as mindfulness, yoga, or deep breathing exercises. If boredom often leads to urges, engaging in a creative hobby, learning a new skill, or participating in a physical activity can provide a meaningful and enjoyable distraction. The key is to find activities that resonate with you and offer genuine satisfaction.

Creating a list of positive alternatives can be a helpful starting point. This list acts as a menu of options you can turn to when faced with an urge. For example, your list might include activities like going for a walk, calling a friend, journaling, listening to music, or cooking a new recipe. Having these options readily available reduces the likelihood of defaulting to the addictive behavior and empowers you to make intentional choices.

Timing and accessibility are critical factors in successfully replacing negative behaviors. Positive alternatives need to be both convenient and immediately accessible, especially in moments of temptation. For instance, if you're trying to replace late-night urges with a relaxing activity, keep a book or journal by your bedside. If physical activity helps you manage stress, ensure you have the necessary gear and a plan for when and where to exercise. The easier it is to engage in the positive behavior, the more likely you are to choose it.

It's also important to recognize that replacing negative behaviors with positive ones is not a one-size-fits-all process. What works for one person may not work for another, so it's important to experiment with different activities and approaches to find what resonates with you. Pay attention to how you feel after trying a new alternative. Does it genuinely satisfy the need or emotion that triggered the urge? If not, consider refining your approach or exploring additional options.

Consistency is key when building new habits. Replacing negative behaviors with positive ones is not just about making a single change; it's about creating patterns that become second nature over time. Start small and focus on repeating the positive behavior regularly. For example, if you decide to replace stress-induced urges with deep breathing, commit to practicing this technique daily, even when you're not feeling stressed. This consistency helps to rewire your brain, making the new behavior more automatic and less reliant on willpower.

In addition to finding specific alternatives, it's helpful to focus on building a lifestyle that supports positive behaviors. This might involve creating a daily routine that includes activities you enjoy, setting goals that align with your values, and surrounding yourself with people who inspire and support you. By fostering an environment that promotes well-being, you make it easier to sustain positive habits and resist the pull of addiction.

Replacing negative behaviors also involves addressing the emotional and mental barriers that might arise during the process. It's natural to feel resistance or doubt, especially when stepping out of your comfort zone or trying something new. Be patient with yourself and approach these moments with curiosity and self-compassion. If you find it challenging to engage in a positive alternative, remind yourself of the reasons you're working toward change and the benefits that come with it.

Celebrating your successes, no matter how small, reinforces your commitment to replacing negative behaviors. Each time you choose a positive alternative over the addictive behavior, you are strengthening your resolve and building momentum. Acknowledge these moments and reflect on how they contribute to your overall progress. This positive reinforcement helps to solidify new habits and reminds you of your ability to take control of your choices.

Finally, remember that replacing negative behaviors with positive ones is a journey, not an instant transformation. Setbacks are a natural part of the process and should not be viewed as failures. Instead, see them as opportunities to learn more about yourself, refine your strategies, and continue moving forward. Each step you take, even if it's imperfect, brings you closer to breaking free from addiction and building a life that reflects your values and aspirations.

By focusing on replacing negative behaviors with positive alternatives, you are not only addressing the immediate challenges of addiction but also creating a foundation for lasting change. These new habits and routines will empower you to navigate life's challenges with resilience and intention, helping you move toward a future of freedom, fulfillment, and self-respect. Each positive choice you make is a step toward reclaiming your life and embracing the person you want to become.

4.3. Dealing with Urges and Relapses

Dealing with urges and relapses is an inevitable part of recovery from addiction to pornography and masturbation. While the goal is to reduce and eventually eliminate these behaviors, it is essential to approach the journey with the understanding that setbacks are not failures but opportunities for growth. The process of overcoming addiction is rarely linear; instead, it involves learning how to navigate the challenges, triggers, and moments of vulnerability that arise along the way. By equipping yourself with strategies to manage urges and respond to relapses constructively, you can build resilience and maintain momentum on your path to recovery.

Urges are the brain's way of seeking the reward it has become accustomed to through repeated patterns of behavior. These moments of craving can feel intense and overwhelming, but they are also temporary. One of the most effective ways to deal with urges is to practice mindfulness and acceptance. Instead of trying to suppress or fight the urge, acknowledge its presence and observe it without judgment. Remind yourself that the urge is a natural part of the recovery process and that it will pass, much like a wave. By allowing the urge to exist without acting on it, you reduce its power over you.

A helpful technique for managing urges is the "pause and reflect" method. When an urge arises, pause for a moment and take a few deep breaths. Use this time to ask yourself questions like, "What am I feeling right now? What triggered this urge? What do I really need in this moment?" This pause creates space between the urge and your response, giving you the opportunity to make a conscious choice rather than reacting impulsively. It also helps you identify the underlying emotions or needs that the urge is attempting to address, such as stress, loneliness, or boredom.

Distraction is another effective strategy for dealing with urges. Engaging in a positive activity that occupies your mind and body can help redirect your attention away from the craving. This might include going for a walk, calling a friend, working on a creative project, or practicing a hobby you enjoy. The key is to choose activities that are readily accessible and engaging enough to shift your focus. Over time, these distractions can become healthy habits that replace the addictive behavior.

Developing a personalized plan for dealing with urges is an important part of recovery. This plan might include a list of activities you can turn to when cravings arise, a set of coping statements or affirmations to remind yourself of your goals, and a support system of people you can reach out to for encouragement. Having this plan in place provides a clear roadmap for navigating moments of temptation and reduces the likelihood of acting on impulses.

Relapses, while discouraging, are a natural part of the recovery journey for many individuals. It's important to approach relapses with compassion and a problem-solving mindset rather than self-criticism. When a relapse occurs, take time to reflect on what led to it. Was there a specific trigger or series of events that contributed to the behavior? Were there warning signs that you overlooked? Understanding the factors that led to the relapse can provide valuable insights for preventing future occurrences.

Instead of dwelling on the relapse as a failure, focus on what you can learn from the experience. Use it as an opportunity to refine your strategies, strengthen your boundaries, and build greater awareness of your triggers. For example, if you realize that certain environments or situations make it difficult to resist urges, you can take proactive steps to avoid or prepare for them in the future. Each relapse is a chance to adjust your approach and grow stronger in your recovery.

It's also important to recognize the progress you've made, even if a relapse feels like a step backward. Recovery is not about achieving perfection; it's about making steady, incremental progress over time. Reflect on the positive changes you've already accomplished, such as reducing the frequency of the behavior, increasing your self-awareness, or developing healthier coping mechanisms. These successes demonstrate your capacity for change and provide motivation to keep moving forward.

Building resilience in the face of urges and relapses involves cultivating a mindset of self-compassion and perseverance. Treat yourself with kindness and understanding, acknowledging that recovery is a challenging process that requires effort and patience. Avoid harsh self-criticism, which can lead to feelings of shame and hopelessness, and instead focus on the steps you can take to get back on track. Remind yourself that every moment is an opportunity to make a different choice and that your commitment to recovery is stronger than any setback.

Having a support system can be invaluable when dealing with urges and relapses. Sharing your struggles with trusted friends, family members, or a recovery group provides encouragement, accountability, and perspective. These connections remind you that you are not alone and that others understand the challenges you face. Reaching out for support during moments of difficulty can help you regain your focus and stay committed to your goals.

Finally, celebrate your resilience and determination to keep moving forward, even in the face of setbacks. Recovery is a journey of growth and transformation, and every step you take—no matter how small—brings you closer to the life you want to create. By learning to navigate urges and respond to relapses with compassion and intention, you are building the skills and mindset needed for lasting change. Each moment of struggle is an opportunity to grow stronger, and each decision to keep going is a testament to your courage and commitment.

4.4. Developing Healthy Coping Mechanisms

Developing healthy coping mechanisms is a fundamental aspect of overcoming addiction to pornography and masturbation. Addiction often serves as a way to manage difficult emotions, stress, or life challenges, providing temporary relief or distraction. However, these behaviors do not address the root causes of distress and often exacerbate feelings of guilt, shame, or dissatisfaction. Building a repertoire of positive coping strategies allows you to confront these underlying issues directly, fostering resilience, emotional balance, and a deeper sense of control over your life.

The first step in developing healthy coping mechanisms is understanding the triggers and emotions that drive your addictive behavior. Reflect on the moments when you feel the strongest urges—what are you experiencing emotionally, mentally, or physically? Common triggers might include stress, loneliness, boredom, frustration, or feelings of inadequacy. By identifying the specific circumstances that lead to these urges, you can begin to match them with alternative responses that address your emotional needs more effectively.

Stress, for example, is a frequent trigger for many individuals. Pornography and masturbation may offer temporary escape from the pressures of work, relationships, or other responsibilities. However, this relief is short-lived and often followed by guilt or regret. To manage stress in a healthier way, consider integrating relaxation techniques into your daily routine. Practices such as deep breathing, progressive muscle relaxation, or mindfulness meditation can help you calm your mind and body, reducing the intensity of stress and improving your ability to handle challenges.

Loneliness and isolation are also common triggers that lead individuals to seek solace in addictive behaviors. These feelings can create a sense of emptiness or disconnection, which pornography and masturbation may temporarily fill. To address loneliness, focus on building meaningful connections with others. This might involve reaching out to friends or family, joining a social group or club, or volunteering in your community. Engaging with others helps to combat feelings of isolation and provides a supportive network that reinforces your recovery journey.

Boredom is another emotional state that often leads to compulsive behavior. The idle moments of unstructured time can create opportunities for old habits to resurface. To counter boredom, fill your schedule with engaging and productive activities that bring you joy or a sense of accomplishment. Pursue hobbies you enjoy, take up a new skill, or set personal goals that challenge and inspire you. By creating a sense of purpose and direction in your life, you reduce the likelihood of turning to addictive behaviors out of boredom.

Frustration and feelings of inadequacy can also play a significant role in sustaining addiction. When faced with challenges or setbacks, it's easy to seek out behaviors that offer immediate gratification. However, this often perpetuates a cycle of avoidance and self-criticism. Developing a growth mindset can help you reframe these moments as opportunities for learning and self-improvement. Instead of viewing setbacks as failures, approach them with curiosity and a willingness to grow. Journaling about your experiences or discussing them with a trusted friend or counselor can provide valuable perspective and support.

In addition to addressing specific triggers, building a daily routine that prioritizes self-care and well-being can help you develop a strong foundation for coping with life's challenges. Regular exercise, for instance, is a powerful way to manage stress, boost mood, and improve overall health. Activities like walking, running, yoga, or swimming release endorphins, which naturally enhance your sense of well-being and reduce cravings for addictive behaviors. Similarly, maintaining a balanced diet and ensuring adequate sleep contribute to emotional stability and resilience.

Engaging in creative or expressive activities is another effective coping mechanism. Artistic pursuits such as painting, writing, music, or dance provide an outlet for processing emotions and exploring your inner world. These activities encourage self-expression and can serve as a healthy distraction during moments of temptation. They also offer a sense of accomplishment and fulfillment, helping to counteract feelings of dissatisfaction or emptiness.

Practicing gratitude is a simple yet impactful way to shift your mindset and build emotional resilience. Take a few moments each day to reflect on the things you are grateful for, whether it's supportive relationships, personal achievements, or small joys in your daily life. Gratitude helps to reframe your perspective, focusing your attention on the positive aspects of your life rather than the challenges. This shift in focus can strengthen your motivation and commitment to recovery.

Learning to sit with uncomfortable emotions is a skill that lies at the heart of healthy coping. Addiction often develops as a way to avoid or numb painful feelings, but true emotional growth comes from facing and processing these emotions. Mindfulness practices can help you observe your thoughts and feelings without becoming overwhelmed by them. By allowing yourself to experience and accept your emotions, you build the capacity to respond to them constructively rather than reacting impulsively.

Having a support system is another crucial element of developing healthy coping mechanisms. Share your struggles and successes with trusted friends, family members, or a support group. These connections provide encouragement, accountability, and perspective, reminding you that you are not alone in your journey. Leaning on others during difficult moments can make a significant difference in your ability to cope and stay committed to your goals.

Finally, remember that building healthy coping mechanisms is a gradual process that requires patience and self-compassion. It's normal to encounter setbacks or challenges along the way, but each effort you make is a step toward greater emotional balance and resilience. Celebrate your progress, no matter how small, and remind yourself that recovery is about growth, not perfection.

By developing and practicing healthy coping mechanisms, you empower yourself to face life's challenges with confidence and intention. These strategies not only help you manage triggers and emotions but also contribute to a richer, more fulfilling life. Each time you choose a healthy coping mechanism over an addictive behavior, you reinforce your commitment to change and move closer to the freedom and self-respect you deserve.

4.5. The Role of Mindfulness in Overcoming Addiction

The role of mindfulness in overcoming addiction to pornography and masturbation is both profound and transformative. Mindfulness, at its core, is the practice of being fully present in the moment, aware of your thoughts, feelings, and bodily sensations without judgment. It allows you to observe your internal experiences with curiosity and acceptance, creating a space between your urges and actions. This practice can help you break the automatic patterns of addictive behavior and develop greater self-awareness and control.

Addiction often thrives on automaticity, where triggers lead to behaviors without conscious thought. Mindfulness disrupts this cycle by encouraging you to pause and observe what is happening within you. When an urge arises, instead of reacting impulsively, you can take a moment to notice the sensations in your body, the thoughts in your mind, and the emotions you're experiencing. By acknowledging these elements without judgment, you reduce their power and create the opportunity to respond intentionally.

One of the most powerful aspects of mindfulness is its ability to help you stay present in moments of discomfort. Addiction often serves as a way to avoid or escape negative emotions, such as stress, loneliness, or frustration. Mindfulness teaches you to sit with these feelings rather than running from them, recognizing that they are temporary and manageable. For example, if you feel an urge driven by boredom or anxiety, mindfulness allows you to observe these feelings without acting on them, trusting that they will pass.

A simple mindfulness technique for managing urges is called "urge surfing." This practice involves visualizing the urge as a wave that rises, peaks, and eventually subsides. Instead of trying to fight or suppress the urge, you ride it like a surfer on a wave, staying present with the sensations and watching as they diminish over time. This approach helps you recognize that urges are not permanent and that you have the strength to endure them without giving in.

Mindfulness also cultivates greater self-awareness, which is essential for understanding the triggers and patterns that sustain addiction. By paying attention to your thoughts and feelings, you can identify the moments when you are most vulnerable to urges and the emotions or situations that drive them. This awareness enables you to anticipate and prepare for these challenges, reducing their impact and empowering you to make healthier choices.

Practicing mindfulness doesn't require a significant time commitment or special equipment. Even a few minutes a day can make a difference. Begin by finding a quiet space where you can sit comfortably and focus on your breath. Pay attention to the sensation of the air entering and leaving your body, letting your breath anchor you in the present moment. When your mind wanders—which it inevitably will—gently bring your attention back to your breath without judgment. This simple exercise can help you develop the skills needed to remain present and grounded, even in the face of strong urges.

Another effective mindfulness practice is the body scan. This involves directing your attention to different parts of your body, noticing any sensations, tension, or discomfort. The body scan can help you become more attuned to the physical manifestations of stress or urges, allowing you to address them with greater awareness. For example, if you notice tightness in your chest or restlessness in your hands, you might take a few deep breaths to release the tension and refocus your energy.

Incorporating mindfulness into your daily routine can also help you develop a greater sense of control and balance. You might practice mindfulness while eating, savoring each bite and noticing the flavors and textures. Or you could try mindful walking, paying attention to the sensation of your feet on the ground and the rhythm of your steps. These practices help you cultivate a habit of presence that extends beyond moments of temptation, enriching your overall sense of well-being.

Mindfulness also fosters self-compassion, an essential quality for navigating the challenges of recovery. Addiction often comes with feelings of guilt, shame, or self-judgment, which can undermine your motivation and make it harder to stay committed to change. By practicing mindfulness, you learn to approach yourself with kindness and understanding, acknowledging your struggles without criticism. This self-compassion creates a supportive internal environment where growth and healing can flourish.

In addition to individual mindfulness practices, consider exploring group activities that incorporate mindfulness, such as yoga or meditation classes. These settings provide a sense of community and accountability, as well as an opportunity to deepen your practice under the guidance of experienced instructors. Engaging with others who share your commitment to mindfulness can also inspire and motivate you on your journey.

The benefits of mindfulness extend far beyond managing addiction. As you cultivate this practice, you may notice improvements in other areas of your life, such as reduced stress, enhanced focus, and greater emotional resilience. These benefits reinforce your recovery by creating a strong foundation of mental and emotional well-being, empowering you to navigate challenges with confidence and clarity.

Ultimately, mindfulness is about reclaiming your ability to choose your actions rather than being controlled by impulses or habits. It teaches you to respond to life's challenges with intention and presence, breaking free from the cycle of addiction and building a life that reflects your values and aspirations. Each moment of mindfulness is a step toward greater freedom, self-respect, and fulfillment. With patience and practice, this simple yet powerful tool can transform your recovery journey and help you embrace a future of balance and purpose.

4.6. Using Technology to Support Recovery

Using technology to support recovery from addiction to pornography and masturbation is a strategic and empowering approach in today's digitally-driven world. While technology can be a source of temptation, it can also be harnessed as a powerful tool for creating accountability, managing triggers, and building new, healthier habits. By intentionally integrating supportive technologies into your recovery plan, you can leverage their benefits to strengthen your commitment and maintain focus on your goals.

One of the most effective ways to use technology for recovery is through the implementation of content filters and blocking software. These tools restrict access to explicit materials, reducing opportunities for impulsive behavior. Apps like Covenant Eyes, Qustodio, or Net Nanny allow you to set boundaries for your internet usage, create accountability by sharing your activity with a trusted partner, or block specific websites entirely. While these tools are not a replacement for personal commitment, they serve as a valuable line of defense against moments of weakness, giving you the space to focus on building healthier habits.

Accountability software is another powerful resource. These programs monitor your online activity and send reports to an accountability partner of your choosing, such as a friend, family member, or mentor. Knowing that someone else is aware of your actions adds a layer of responsibility and can deter you from engaging in addictive behaviors. This transparency creates a collaborative approach to recovery, where you feel supported rather than isolated in your efforts.

Scheduling and habit-tracking apps can also play a vital role in your recovery journey. Apps like Habitica, Streaks, or Done allow you to set goals, track your progress, and receive reminders to stay on track. For instance, you can use these tools to monitor your streaks of abstinence, set reminders to practice mindfulness, or schedule activities that replace negative behaviors with positive ones. Celebrating milestones within these apps reinforces your achievements and provides motivation to keep moving forward.

Meditation and mindfulness apps, such as Headspace, Calm, or Insight Timer, can support emotional regulation and self-awareness—two critical elements of recovery. These apps offer guided meditations, breathing exercises, and relaxation techniques designed to help you manage stress, reduce anxiety, and remain present in the moment. Incorporating daily mindfulness practices through these tools can help you navigate urges and build resilience against triggers.

If you find that boredom or idle time often leads to urges, consider using technology to engage in productive or enjoyable activities. Educational platforms like Duolingo, Skillshare, or MasterClass provide opportunities to learn new skills, explore hobbies, or deepen your knowledge in areas of interest. Streaming services that offer inspiring or educational content can also serve as a constructive alternative to unstructured browsing. By intentionally filling your free time with enriching activities, you reduce the likelihood of falling into old patterns.

Digital support groups and online communities are another valuable resource for recovery. Platforms like Reddit (e.g., r/NoFap), Quit Porn Community, or other forums offer a space to connect with individuals who share similar goals and challenges. Engaging in these communities provides a sense of belonging, encouragement, and accountability. Sharing your experiences and learning from others can inspire new strategies and reinforce your commitment to change.

Setting up technology-free zones or times can also help you create a healthier relationship with your devices. Designate specific areas in your home—such as the bedroom or dining area—as screen-free zones, or establish times during the day when you disconnect entirely. These boundaries reduce the likelihood of encountering triggers and encourage you to focus on offline activities that promote well-being, such as reading, exercising, or spending time with loved ones.

Personalized digital tools, such as journaling apps or mood trackers, can help you gain deeper insight into your recovery journey. Writing down your thoughts and feelings in a secure digital journal allows you to track patterns, reflect on progress, and identify triggers. Similarly, mood-tracking apps like Daylio or Moodpath can help you monitor your emotional states over time, revealing connections between your feelings and behaviors.

For those who prefer one-on-one guidance, teletherapy platforms such as BetterHelp, Talkspace, or other online counseling services provide access to professional support from the comfort of your home. These services offer flexible scheduling, confidentiality, and a wide range of therapists who specialize in addiction recovery. Regular sessions with a therapist can provide valuable insights, coping strategies, and emotional support tailored to your unique needs.

Lastly, setting intentional limits on your overall technology use can help you build a more balanced and mindful lifestyle. Features like screen time trackers on your smartphone or apps like Freedom or StayFocusd can help you monitor and manage your time online. By reducing excessive screen time, you free up energy and attention for activities that align with your recovery goals and personal values.

Using technology to support recovery is about reclaiming its role in your life as a tool for empowerment rather than a source of distraction or temptation. By intentionally integrating supportive technologies, you create an environment that aligns with your goals and reinforces your commitment to change. Each time you use these tools effectively, you take a step toward breaking free from addictive patterns and building a life of balance, purpose, and fulfillment. Embrace the positive potential of technology as a partner in your recovery, and let it guide you toward the freedom and self-respect you deserve.

Chapter 5: Rebuilding Your Life

Rebuilding your life after addiction to pornography and masturbation is about more than simply stopping the behavior. It is a journey of rediscovery, healing, and growth. While the early stages of recovery often focus on breaking harmful patterns and managing triggers, the next phase involves creating a life that aligns with your values, aspirations, and sense of self-worth. This chapter is dedicated to helping you rebuild your life in a way that fosters confidence, connection, and fulfillment.

Addiction often leaves behind a sense of emptiness or disconnection, not only from others but also from yourself. Rebuilding your life requires addressing these feelings by nurturing self-esteem, cultivating meaningful relationships, and rediscovering passions and interests that bring you joy. It's about filling the spaces left by addiction with positive, life-affirming pursuits that contribute to your overall well-being.

This process involves intentional effort and a willingness to explore new possibilities. As you rebuild, you will face opportunities to challenge limiting beliefs, strengthen your sense of identity, and reestablish trust with yourself and those around you. Each step forward, no matter how small, is a chance to redefine your relationship with yourself and your world, creating a foundation for lasting change.

Rebuilding your life also means learning to embrace vulnerability and intimacy in healthier ways. Addiction often distorts perceptions of relationships and intimacy, creating barriers to genuine connection. By addressing these distortions and fostering emotional openness, you can develop stronger, more authentic bonds with others. This chapter will explore how to navigate these changes and build relationships that support your growth.

This stage of recovery is about more than just "moving on"—it's about moving forward with intention and purpose. It's a chance to reclaim your time, energy, and potential, directing them toward goals and aspirations that resonate with your values. Rebuilding your life is not just about leaving addiction behind; it's about embracing the freedom to create a future that reflects who you truly want to be. Let this chapter guide you on the path to restoring confidence, rebuilding connections, and living with purpose and fulfillment.

5.1. Restoring Self-Esteem and Confidence

Restoring self-esteem and confidence is one of the most empowering aspects of recovery from addiction to pornography and masturbation. Addiction often leaves individuals with feelings of guilt, shame, and inadequacy, eroding their sense of self-worth over time. As you move forward in your recovery journey, rebuilding your self-esteem is not just about healing the wounds left by addiction—it's about rediscovering your inherent value, embracing your strengths, and fostering a positive, compassionate relationship with yourself.

The first step in restoring self-esteem is to shift the way you perceive yourself. Addiction can create a narrative of failure or weakness, where you define yourself by past mistakes or struggles. Breaking free from this narrative requires recognizing that addiction does not define who you are. It is a condition that you are working to overcome, not a reflection of your character or worth. Remind yourself that recovery is a courageous and commendable journey, and the effort you are putting into change speaks volumes about your resilience and strength.

Practicing self-compassion is essential in this process. Self-compassion involves treating yourself with kindness, understanding, and forgiveness, especially during moments of struggle or setback. Instead of criticizing yourself for past behaviors or perceived shortcomings, acknowledge your efforts and celebrate the progress you've made. Recovery is not about perfection; it's about growth, and each step you take toward a healthier life is a testament to your determination and capability.

Setting small, achievable goals can be a powerful way to rebuild confidence. These goals might involve daily habits, such as practicing mindfulness, engaging in physical activity, or dedicating time to a hobby or skill. Each goal you accomplish reinforces your belief in your ability to create positive change and take control of your life. Over time, these small successes build momentum, gradually restoring your sense of competence and self-efficacy.

Reflecting on your strengths and accomplishments is another important practice. Addiction often narrows your focus, making it easy to overlook the qualities and achievements that make you who you are. Take time to identify your strengths—whether it's your creativity, empathy, determination, or problem-solving skills—and consider how these attributes have supported you throughout your life. Acknowledge the achievements you're proud of, no matter how big or small, and let them remind you of your potential.

Surrounding yourself with supportive and affirming relationships can also play a significant role in restoring self-esteem. Seek out individuals who uplift and encourage you, and who recognize your worth beyond the struggles you've faced. Sharing your journey with trusted friends, family members, or support groups provides not only validation but also a sense of connection and belonging. These relationships remind you that you are valued and appreciated, reinforcing your self-esteem.

Rebuilding confidence often involves stepping out of your comfort zone and taking on new challenges. These challenges don't need to be monumental; even small acts of courage, such as trying a new activity, initiating a conversation, or setting a boundary, can boost your confidence. Each time you take a step into the unknown and succeed, you reinforce your belief in your abilities and expand your sense of what is possible.

It's also important to address and reframe negative self-talk. The internal dialogue that accompanies addiction can be harsh and unforgiving, filled with self-criticism and doubt. Challenge these thoughts by replacing them with affirmations or reminders of your worth and progress. For example, instead of thinking, "I'll never overcome this," remind yourself, "I'm making progress every day, and I have the strength to keep going." Over time, cultivating a positive inner voice helps to rebuild your self-esteem from within.

Engaging in acts of self-care is another vital component of restoring self-esteem. Taking care of your physical, emotional, and mental health sends a message to yourself that you are worthy of love and attention. This might involve prioritizing sleep, eating nourishing meals, exercising regularly, or dedicating time to relaxation and reflection. These acts of care not only improve your overall well-being but also reinforce your sense of self-worth.

Volunteering or contributing to your community can also enhance self-esteem by giving you a sense of purpose and connection. Helping others allows you to focus on the positive impact you can have in the world, shifting attention away from feelings of inadequacy or guilt.

Whether it's mentoring someone, participating in a community project, or simply being a supportive friend, these acts of kindness remind you of your value and capability.

Restoring self-esteem and confidence is a gradual and ongoing process, and it's important to celebrate the progress you make along the way. Recovery is a journey of self-discovery, where you learn not only to let go of the past but also to embrace the person you are becoming. Each act of self-compassion, each step toward a goal, and each moment of self-awareness contributes to rebuilding your sense of self-worth.

Ultimately, restoring self-esteem and confidence is about reclaiming your identity and recognizing that you are more than your struggles. It's about embracing your strengths, celebrating your progress, and believing in your ability to create a fulfilling and purposeful life. As you continue to grow and heal, you will discover that confidence and self-esteem are not just the results of recovery—they are the foundation for building a life of freedom, connection, and self-respect.

5.2. Reconnecting with Real-Life Relationships

Reconnecting with real-life relationships is one of the most rewarding and transformative aspects of recovery from addiction to pornography and masturbation. Addiction often creates a sense of isolation, driving a wedge between you and the people who matter most in your life. Whether through secrecy, guilt, or emotional withdrawal, addiction can strain even the closest connections. Rebuilding these relationships and forming new, meaningful bonds is not only possible but also essential for long-term recovery and personal growth.

The first step in reconnecting with others is acknowledging the impact addiction may have had on your relationships. This is not about dwelling on guilt or blame but about understanding the ways in which your behavior may have created distance or hurt. Reflecting on these dynamics with honesty and compassion allows you to approach the process of reconnection with greater awareness and humility. It's important to remember that repairing relationships is a journey that requires time, patience, and mutual effort.

Opening lines of communication is a critical part of reconnecting. Addiction often thrives in secrecy, but rebuilding trust and intimacy requires transparency. Consider reaching out to the people who have been affected by your behavior—whether they are partners, family members, or close friends—and sharing your commitment to recovery. This doesn't mean disclosing every detail but rather expressing your desire to reconnect and work on the relationship. Be prepared to listen to their feelings and perspectives, even if they are difficult to hear. Genuine communication lays the foundation for rebuilding trust.

In some cases, reconnecting may involve offering an apology or taking responsibility for past actions. Apologies should be heartfelt and focused on acknowledging the impact of your behavior rather than making excuses or seeking forgiveness. For example, you might say, "I realize my actions have hurt you, and I'm deeply sorry for the pain I've caused. I'm committed to making changes and rebuilding our relationship." Taking accountability demonstrates sincerity and a willingness to grow, fostering an environment where healing can begin.

Rebuilding trust is a gradual process that requires consistent effort and reliability. Trust is not restored through words alone but through actions that demonstrate your commitment to change. This might involve keeping promises, being present and attentive, and showing consideration for the other person's needs and feelings. Over time, these actions help to repair the fractures caused by addiction and create a stronger, more stable foundation for the relationship.

Engaging in shared activities is another powerful way to reconnect with loved ones. Addiction often monopolizes time and energy, leaving little room for meaningful interactions. By participating in activities together—such as cooking, hiking, or playing games—you create opportunities to rebuild connection and create positive memories. These shared experiences foster a sense of closeness and remind you both of the joy and value of the relationship.

For those in romantic relationships, reconnecting may involve addressing the ways addiction has impacted intimacy and trust. Addiction to pornography, in particular, can create unrealistic expectations or distortions about physical and emotional closeness, leading to misunderstandings or feelings of inadequacy. Open and honest conversations about your needs, boundaries, and goals for the relationship are essential for rebuilding intimacy. Consider seeking the guidance of a therapist or counselor to navigate these discussions and strengthen your connection.

As you reconnect with others, it's important to recognize that not every relationship may be salvageable or healthy to pursue. Some connections may have been built on dynamics that no longer align with your values or recovery goals. In these cases, it's okay to let go and focus on relationships that support your growth and well-being. Surrounding yourself with people who encourage and inspire you is vital for maintaining a positive and supportive environment.

Building new relationships can also be an important part of recovery. Addiction often leads to isolation, but forming new connections provides a sense of belonging and community. Consider joining groups or organizations that align with your interests, such as a hobby club, sports team, or volunteer group. These settings offer opportunities to meet like-minded individuals and foster meaningful relationships that enrich your life.

Reconnecting with real-life relationships also involves setting healthy boundaries. Recovery requires prioritizing your well-being, and this sometimes means establishing limits with people or situations that trigger stress or temptation. Boundaries are not about shutting people out but about creating a space where you can thrive. Communicate your boundaries clearly and respectfully, and remember that protecting your recovery is an act of self-respect and care.

Practicing vulnerability is another important aspect of rebuilding relationships. Addiction often creates a shield of emotional detachment, making it difficult to share your true self with others. Allowing yourself to be open and authentic—whether by sharing your struggles, hopes, or fears—fosters deeper connections and strengthens the bonds of trust and intimacy. Vulnerability is a sign of courage and a key ingredient in meaningful relationships.

Finally, give yourself and others grace during the process of reconnection. Healing relationships takes time, and progress may not always be linear. Be patient with yourself as you navigate these changes, and extend the same understanding to the people in your life. Recovery is a journey of mutual growth, where both you and your loved ones can learn, heal, and build a brighter future together.

Reconnecting with real-life relationships is about more than mending what was broken—it's about creating stronger, more authentic connections that enrich your life and support your recovery. These relationships remind you of your inherent worth and provide a source of encouragement, love, and belonging. By fostering these connections, you not only rebuild the social fabric of your life but also rediscover the joy and fulfillment that come from meaningful human connection.

5.3. Cultivating Healthy Intimacy

Cultivating healthy intimacy is an essential part of recovery from addiction to pornography and masturbation. Addiction often distorts perceptions of intimacy, replacing genuine connection with superficial or unrealistic representations. Over time, this can erode your ability to experience and nurture authentic closeness with others. Rebuilding intimacy involves re-learning how to connect deeply, both emotionally and physically, in ways that align with your values and foster meaningful relationships. This process is not only about healing the damage caused by addiction but also about rediscovering the joy and fulfillment that come from genuine intimacy.

Healthy intimacy begins with self-awareness and self-acceptance. Before you can connect deeply with others, it's important to develop a strong relationship with yourself. Addiction often creates feelings of shame or self-criticism that can act as barriers to intimacy. By practicing self-compassion and recognizing your inherent worth, you can begin to approach relationships from a place of confidence and authenticity. Accepting yourself, flaws and all, creates the foundation for sharing your true self with others.

Emotional intimacy is a key aspect of healthy relationships. It involves being open and vulnerable, sharing your thoughts, feelings, and experiences with another person. For many recovering from addiction, vulnerability can feel uncomfortable or risky, especially if past experiences have led to rejection or hurt. However, cultivating emotional intimacy requires a willingness to take these risks, trusting that meaningful connection is worth the effort. Start by opening up gradually, sharing your feelings with someone you trust, and allowing the relationship to deepen over time.

One of the challenges in cultivating healthy intimacy is addressing the unrealistic expectations or misconceptions about relationships that addiction may have fostered. Pornography, in particular, often portrays intimacy as purely physical, devoid of emotional connection, or based on unattainable ideals. These distorted views can create dissatisfaction or unrealistic standards in real-life relationships. To counter this, it's important to approach intimacy with a sense of curiosity and openness, embracing the imperfections and complexities that make genuine connection so meaningful.

Physical intimacy is another important dimension of healthy relationships, but it should always be built on a foundation of trust, respect, and mutual consent. For those in romantic partnerships, rebuilding physical intimacy may involve addressing any lingering feelings of insecurity or mistrust caused by addiction. Open and honest communication with your partner is essential, allowing both of you to express your needs, boundaries, and concerns. If these conversations feel challenging, consider seeking the guidance of a therapist or counselor to navigate them in a supportive and constructive way.

Relearning physical intimacy also involves being present and attentive in the moment. Addiction can often create a sense of detachment, where physical interactions become transactional or disconnected from emotion. By practicing mindfulness during moments of physical closeness—focusing on the sensations, emotions, and connection you feel—you can deepen your experience of intimacy and strengthen the bond with your partner.

For those who are not currently in a romantic relationship, cultivating healthy intimacy might involve building closer connections with friends or family members. Intimacy is not limited to romantic or physical relationships; it can also be found in the emotional bonds you share with loved ones. Prioritize spending quality time with people who uplift and support you, engaging in meaningful conversations and shared experiences. These interactions remind you of the richness and depth of human connection, reinforcing your commitment to fostering healthy relationships.

Setting boundaries is another crucial aspect of cultivating healthy intimacy. Boundaries help protect your well-being and ensure that your relationships are built on mutual respect. For example, you might set boundaries around how and when you engage with others, or establish limits on conversations or behaviors that feel triggering or unhealthy. Communicating these boundaries clearly and assertively helps create a safe space for intimacy to flourish.

Developing patience is also important when rebuilding intimacy. Healing takes time, both for yourself and for your relationships. Be gentle with yourself as you navigate this process, and understand that intimacy cannot be rushed or forced. Allow your connections to grow naturally, focusing on building trust and understanding rather than striving for immediate closeness. By giving yourself and others the time and space needed to heal, you create a more authentic and lasting foundation for intimacy.

Engaging in activities that promote emotional and physical connection can also support your efforts to cultivate healthy intimacy. For example, spending time together without distractions, engaging in shared hobbies, or practicing partner-based exercises such as yoga or dance can strengthen your bond and foster a sense of closeness. These activities encourage you to be present with one another, deepening your understanding and appreciation of the relationship.

Ultimately, cultivating healthy intimacy is about creating relationships that are authentic, respectful, and mutually fulfilling. It's about moving away from the superficial or transactional dynamics of addiction and embracing the richness of genuine connection. As you rebuild intimacy in your life, you will discover not only the joy of deeper relationships but also a renewed sense of self-worth and purpose. Healthy intimacy is a powerful antidote to the isolation and disconnection that addiction creates, offering a path to healing, growth, and enduring fulfillment.

5.4. Pursuing New Hobbies and Passions

Pursuing new hobbies and passions is an integral part of rebuilding your life after addiction to pornography and masturbation. Addiction often consumes time and energy that could otherwise be spent exploring your interests, developing skills, or engaging in activities that bring joy and fulfillment. As you progress in your recovery, discovering and embracing new hobbies can help fill the void left by addiction, providing a sense of purpose, creativity, and connection.

One of the most transformative aspects of pursuing new hobbies is the opportunity to reconnect with your authentic self. Addiction often narrows your focus and suppresses your natural curiosity, leaving little room for self-expression or exploration. By engaging in activities that resonate with your interests and values, you can begin to rediscover who you are outside the framework of addiction. This process fosters self-awareness and personal growth, helping you build a stronger, more positive sense of identity.

Exploring new hobbies is also an effective way to counteract boredom, one of the common triggers for addictive behavior. Boredom can create a sense of restlessness or dissatisfaction, leading you to seek out familiar but unhealthy ways to pass the time. Introducing hobbies into your daily routine not only keeps you occupied but also provides meaningful and enjoyable alternatives to the behaviors you're working to overcome. Whether it's learning to play an instrument, experimenting with cooking, or gardening, these activities offer a productive outlet for your energy and creativity.

Physical hobbies, such as sports, hiking, or yoga, can be particularly beneficial during recovery. Physical activity releases endorphins, which naturally boost mood and reduce stress, helping to counteract the emotional triggers that often lead to addictive behaviors. Additionally, physical hobbies promote overall health and well-being, reinforcing your commitment to self-care. Activities that involve movement also provide a sense of accomplishment and progress, which can be motivating and empowering as you rebuild your life.

Creative pursuits are another valuable avenue for personal expression and healing. Art, writing, music, or crafting allow you to channel your emotions into tangible creations, offering a sense of catharsis and achievement. These hobbies provide a safe space to explore your feelings and experiences, helping you process the challenges of recovery while celebrating your growth. The act of creating something meaningful reinforces your ability to bring positive change into your life.

Social hobbies, such as joining a club, volunteering, or participating in group activities, are also excellent for fostering connection and combating the isolation that addiction often creates. Building relationships with people who share your interests helps you form a supportive community and reminds you of the joy and fulfillment that come from meaningful interactions. Social hobbies also provide opportunities to develop communication skills, practice vulnerability, and strengthen your sense of belonging.

If you're unsure where to start, think back to activities you enjoyed in the past but may have set aside due to addiction or other life circumstances. Reconnecting with these interests can reignite your passion and provide a sense of continuity with your personal history. Alternatively, consider trying something completely new and outside your comfort zone. Exploring unfamiliar activities can be both exciting and empowering, giving you the chance to challenge yourself and discover hidden talents.

To make hobbies a lasting part of your life, it's helpful to incorporate them into your routine. Set aside dedicated time for your chosen activities, treating them as a priority rather than an afterthought. Consistency not only helps you build skills and confidence but also reinforces the positive habits you're developing. Over time, these hobbies become an integral part of your daily life, contributing to your overall sense of purpose and well-being.

It's also important to approach hobbies with a sense of curiosity and enjoyment rather than pressure or perfectionism. The goal is not to excel or achieve mastery overnight but to engage in activities that bring you happiness and fulfillment. Allow yourself to make mistakes, explore different options, and simply enjoy the process of learning and creating. Recovery is about progress, not perfection, and hobbies are a space where you can celebrate your growth without judgment.

Pursuing new hobbies and passions also provides an opportunity to set and achieve goals, which can be incredibly motivating during recovery. These goals might involve completing a project, mastering a skill, or participating in an event. Achieving these milestones reinforces your belief in your abilities and reminds you of the rewards of dedication and effort. Each accomplishment, no matter how small, is a step toward rebuilding your confidence and creating a life that aligns with your values.

Finally, hobbies remind you that life is about more than overcoming addiction—it's about discovering and embracing the things that make life meaningful. They allow you to focus on what you're moving toward rather than what you're leaving behind, shifting your perspective from one of limitation to one of possibility. By pursuing new hobbies and passions, you reclaim your time and energy, directing them toward activities that enrich your life and reflect the person you are becoming.

Incorporating hobbies into your recovery journey is not just about filling time; it's about creating a life that feels vibrant, purposeful, and fulfilling. These activities provide a sense of joy, achievement, and connection that strengthens your commitment to change. As you explore and embrace your interests, you'll discover that pursuing new hobbies is not just an act of recovery—it's an act of self-discovery, empowerment, and celebration.

5.5. The Role of Physical Fitness and Nutrition in Recovery

The role of physical fitness and nutrition in recovery from addiction to pornography and masturbation is profoundly impactful, addressing both the physical and psychological dimensions of healing. Addiction often takes a toll on the body and mind, contributing to feelings of lethargy, stress, and disconnection. By prioritizing physical fitness and adopting healthy nutritional habits, you can support your body's natural healing processes, boost your energy levels, and cultivate a sense of well-being that reinforces your recovery journey.

Physical fitness serves as a powerful tool for managing the stress and emotional triggers that often accompany addiction. Exercise releases endorphins, the body's natural "feel-good" chemicals, which help to elevate mood and reduce anxiety. Regular physical activity also improves sleep quality, enhances focus, and increases self-confidence, all of which are essential for sustaining long-term recovery. Whether it's running, swimming, yoga, weightlifting, or even a daily walk, incorporating movement into your routine provides a constructive outlet for stress and pent-up energy.

One of the most significant benefits of physical fitness is its ability to combat the lethargy and lack of motivation that can linger during recovery. Addiction often creates cycles of inactivity or escapism, which can leave you feeling drained or disconnected from your body. Exercise reverses this by reawakening your physical vitality and helping you reconnect with your body in a positive and empowering way. Over time, as your strength and stamina increase, so does your confidence in your ability to overcome challenges and achieve your goals.

The key to integrating physical fitness into your recovery journey is finding activities that you enjoy and that align with your interests and lifestyle. This ensures that exercise becomes a sustainable and enjoyable part of your daily life rather than a chore or obligation. Experiment with different types of movement to discover what resonates with you—whether it's team sports, hiking in nature, dance classes, or solo workouts at the gym. The more you look forward to your chosen activities, the easier it will be to maintain consistency.

Nutrition plays an equally vital role in supporting recovery, as the food you consume directly impacts your physical and mental health. Addiction often leads to neglect of proper nutrition, resulting in imbalances that can affect mood, energy levels, and overall well-being. Rebuilding your health through mindful eating helps to restore balance and provides your body with the nutrients it needs to thrive.

A balanced diet rich in whole, unprocessed foods is the foundation of good nutrition. Focus on incorporating plenty of fruits, vegetables, lean proteins, whole grains, and healthy fats into your meals. These foods provide essential vitamins, minerals, and antioxidants that support brain function, stabilize mood, and boost energy. For example, omega-3 fatty acids found in fish, walnuts, and flaxseeds are known to enhance cognitive function and reduce symptoms of depression, making them particularly beneficial during recovery.

Hydration is another critical aspect of nutrition that is often overlooked. Drinking plenty of water throughout the day helps to maintain energy levels, improve focus, and support overall bodily functions. Dehydration can exacerbate feelings of fatigue or irritability, so make it a priority to stay well-hydrated as part of your self-care routine.

Avoiding or minimizing certain substances can also aid in your recovery. Excessive caffeine, sugar, and processed foods can lead to energy crashes and mood swings, making it harder to stay focused and motivated. While it's not necessary to eliminate these entirely, being mindful of their effects on your body and moderating your intake can improve your overall sense of balance and stability.

Incorporating mindful eating practices can deepen your connection to the food you consume and help you make healthier choices. Mindful eating involves paying attention to the taste, texture, and aroma of your meals, as well as listening to your body's hunger and fullness cues. This practice encourages you to savor each bite and develop a greater appreciation for nourishing your body. It also reduces the likelihood of emotional or mindless eating, which can sometimes replace addictive behaviors.

The synergy between physical fitness and nutrition amplifies their individual benefits, creating a powerful foundation for recovery. For example, regular exercise increases your body's need for nutrients, making it easier to adopt healthier eating habits. Conversely, a balanced diet provides the energy and stamina needed to sustain physical activity. Together, these practices reinforce a cycle of positive change that supports both your body and mind.

As you integrate fitness and nutrition into your recovery journey, it's important to set realistic goals and celebrate your progress. Start with small, achievable steps, such as taking a daily walk or incorporating one healthy meal into your routine. Over time, build on these habits to create a sustainable lifestyle that aligns with your values and aspirations. Remember that consistency is more important than perfection; even small changes can have a significant impact when practiced regularly.

Physical fitness and nutrition also serve as a reminder of your agency and ability to care for yourself. Addiction often creates a sense of disconnection from your body, but these practices allow you to reclaim that connection in a way that feels empowering and affirming. Each workout, healthy meal, or moment of self-care is a testament to your commitment to recovery and your desire to build a life that reflects your full potential.

Incorporating physical fitness and nutrition into your recovery journey is about more than improving your health—it's about nurturing a sense of vitality, strength, and self-respect. These practices provide a solid foundation for emotional resilience and help you build momentum toward a life of balance and fulfillment. By prioritizing your body's needs, you are not only supporting your recovery but also creating a future where you feel energized, confident, and ready to embrace all that life has to offer.

5.6. Long-Term Strategies for Maintaining Freedom

Long-term strategies for maintaining freedom from addiction to pornography and masturbation are essential for sustaining the progress you've made and ensuring that the changes you've worked so hard to achieve remain part of your life. Recovery is not a single event but a lifelong commitment to growth, self-awareness, and intentionality. As you move beyond the initial stages of breaking free from addiction, establishing habits and practices that reinforce your resilience and support your values is crucial for maintaining lasting freedom.

One of the most important strategies for long-term success is fostering self-awareness. Addiction often thrives in the absence of reflection, where automatic behaviors dominate decision-making. Continuing to cultivate self-awareness allows you to recognize potential triggers, identify moments of vulnerability, and respond to challenges with intention rather than reactivity. Practices like journaling, mindfulness, and regular self-reflection help you stay attuned to your thoughts and emotions, giving you the tools to navigate life's ups and downs with clarity and purpose.

Consistency is key when it comes to maintaining freedom from addiction. The habits and routines you've established during your recovery journey should remain an integral part of your life. Whether it's engaging in physical activity, practicing mindfulness, or dedicating time to hobbies and relationships, these practices provide structure and stability, reinforcing your commitment to a healthier, more fulfilling lifestyle. Consistency doesn't mean perfection—life will inevitably bring challenges—but it does mean returning to these practices even when things feel difficult.

Setting long-term goals can also help you maintain focus and motivation. These goals might involve personal growth, career aspirations, or relationships, and they provide a sense of direction that keeps you moving forward. When you're working toward something meaningful, you're less likely to be tempted by old habits that no longer serve you. Break your goals into smaller, actionable steps, and celebrate your progress along the way. Achieving these milestones reinforces your belief in your ability to create a life that reflects your values and aspirations.

Accountability continues to play a vital role in sustaining recovery. Sharing your journey with trusted friends, family members, or a support group provides encouragement and perspective, as well as a sense of responsibility. Knowing that others are invested in your success can motivate you to stay committed, even during moments of doubt or challenge. Regular check-ins with your accountability partners can help you stay on track and provide a safe space to discuss your experiences.

Learning to navigate setbacks with resilience and self-compassion is another critical component of maintaining long-term freedom. Setbacks are a natural part of any recovery journey and do not erase the progress you've made. Instead of viewing them as failures, approach them as opportunities to learn and grow. Reflect on what led to the setback, identify any patterns or triggers, and use that insight to refine your strategies. Treat yourself with kindness and understanding, reminding yourself that recovery is about persistence and progress, not perfection.

Developing a strong support network is essential for maintaining freedom from addiction. Surround yourself with people who uplift and inspire you, and who share your commitment to personal growth and well-being. These relationships provide a source of encouragement and connection, reminding you that you are not alone in your journey. Consider joining a community or group that aligns with your values, whether it's a recovery group, a hobby club, or a spiritual or mindfulness-based organization.

Continuing to expand your understanding of addiction and personal growth can also strengthen your recovery. Reading books, attending workshops, or seeking therapy can deepen your knowledge and provide new insights and tools for navigating life's challenges. Personal growth is a lifelong process, and staying curious and open to learning ensures that you remain engaged with your recovery and the possibilities for your future.

Building a balanced and fulfilling lifestyle is perhaps the most effective long-term strategy for maintaining freedom. When your life is rich with purpose, joy, and connection, there is less room for the habits and behaviors associated with addiction. Focus on nurturing all aspects of your well-being, including your physical, emotional, social, and spiritual health. This might involve exploring new interests, cultivating meaningful relationships, or dedicating time to self-care and reflection.

Regularly revisiting your values and motivations is another way to sustain your recovery. Remind yourself why you chose to break free from addiction and what you've gained through your journey. Reflect on the person you are becoming and the life you are building, and use these reflections to reinforce your commitment to staying on this path. Keeping a written reminder of your values and goals can serve as a powerful anchor during challenging moments.

Finally, celebrate your progress and achievements. Recovery is a remarkable accomplishment, and acknowledging how far you've come helps to reinforce your belief in your ability to maintain freedom. Take time to reflect on the positive changes in your life, whether it's improved relationships, greater self-confidence, or a renewed sense of purpose. Celebrating these milestones not only honors your efforts but also provides motivation to keep moving forward.

Long-term recovery is about more than simply avoiding old habits —it's about creating a life that feels rich, meaningful, and aligned with your true self. By continuing to prioritize self-awareness, consistency, accountability, and balance, you can maintain the freedom you've worked so hard to achieve. Each day is an opportunity to grow, explore, and embrace the possibilities of a life free from addiction, where your choices reflect your values and your actions align with your aspirations.

Chapter 6: Moving Forward

Moving forward after overcoming addiction to pornography and masturbation is about embracing the freedom and possibilities that come with a renewed sense of self. Recovery is not just a process of leaving something behind—it's a journey of stepping into a new chapter of life with confidence, purpose, and resilience. This final stage is about solidifying the changes you've made, preventing relapse, and cultivating habits and perspectives that allow you to thrive long-term.

As you look ahead, it's important to recognize the progress you've made and the strength you've shown throughout your journey. Recovery has likely required you to confront difficult emotions, reevaluate your values, and make significant changes in your daily life. These efforts are not just signs of growth—they are evidence of your capacity to create lasting, meaningful transformation. Moving forward means honoring that progress and building upon it to create a life that aligns with your true self.

This chapter focuses on the tools and strategies that will help you sustain your freedom, deepen your self-awareness, and continue growing as an individual. It addresses how to live without the shame or stigma that addiction might have left behind, how to stay vigilant against potential setbacks, and how to develop a healthy and positive relationship with your sexuality. It also encourages you to consider how your journey can inspire and support others, offering a sense of purpose beyond your personal recovery.

Moving forward also involves embracing the inevitable challenges and uncertainties of life with resilience and grace. While the journey of recovery equips you with the skills to navigate these moments, it's important to remain adaptable and open to learning. Each new experience, whether joyful or difficult, is an opportunity to grow and reaffirm your commitment to living authentically.

This chapter invites you to look beyond the confines of addiction and imagine the life you want to create. It's a life of self-respect, connection, and fulfillment—a life where your choices reflect your values, and your actions are driven by purpose rather than compulsion. As you move forward, remember that recovery is not just an ending but a beginning, offering the freedom to live fully, love deeply, and explore the vast potential within yourself. Let this final chapter guide you as you step boldly into the future, carrying with you the strength and wisdom you've gained along the way.

6.1. Living Without Shame or Stigma

Living without shame or stigma after overcoming addiction to pornography and masturbation is one of the most liberating aspects of recovery. Shame often accompanies addiction, feeding into cycles of secrecy, self-criticism, and emotional isolation. It's a heavy burden that not only weighs on your self-esteem but also reinforces the behaviors you're striving to leave behind. Moving beyond shame is not only about reclaiming your self-worth but also about embracing a life where your past no longer defines you.

To live without shame, it's crucial to understand the difference between guilt and shame. Guilt arises from recognizing that a specific action was wrong or harmful, whereas shame goes deeper, leading you to believe that *you* are fundamentally flawed or unworthy. While guilt can be constructive, prompting reflection and change, shame is destructive, undermining your confidence and sense of self. Recovery involves letting go of shame and focusing on the growth and progress you've made.

A powerful way to overcome shame is by reframing your perspective on addiction. Rather than viewing it as a moral failing, see it as a challenge you've faced and are actively working to overcome. Everyone encounters struggles in life, and your journey to recovery is a testament to your strength and resilience. By shifting the narrative, you transform feelings of inadequacy into a sense of accomplishment for the effort and courage you've shown.

Practicing self-compassion is an essential part of shedding shame. Speak to yourself with kindness and understanding, especially when reflecting on your past. Acknowledge that you, like everyone else, are human and imperfect. Mistakes are a natural part of growth, and they do not diminish your worth or potential. By treating yourself with the same empathy you would offer a friend, you create a supportive inner dialogue that fosters healing and self-acceptance.

Connecting with others who understand your journey can also help dissolve feelings of shame. Addiction often thrives in secrecy, but sharing your experiences with trusted individuals—whether friends, family, or a support group—provides validation and reduces the sense of isolation. When others listen without judgment and acknowledge your efforts, it becomes easier to see yourself through a more compassionate lens. These connections remind you that you are not alone and that your worth extends far beyond your past struggles.

Releasing shame also involves challenging societal stigma. Cultural attitudes toward addiction, particularly pornography and masturbation, are often steeped in judgment and misunderstanding. These stigmas can exacerbate feelings of guilt and fear, making it difficult to seek help or talk openly about your experiences. Educating yourself about the science of addiction and its widespread nature can help you recognize that you are not an anomaly but part of a larger conversation about human behavior and resilience. Advocacy and raising awareness, even in small ways, can empower you and contribute to changing the narrative for others.

Forgiveness is another key step in moving beyond shame. This includes forgiving yourself for past actions and, where necessary, seeking or granting forgiveness in your relationships. Self-forgiveness allows you to release the emotional weight of guilt and regret, freeing you to focus on the present and future. It's not about excusing harmful behavior but about acknowledging your growth and the efforts you're making to live in alignment with your values.

Living without shame also means embracing your new identity as a person in recovery. You are not defined by your addiction but by the choices you make and the person you are becoming. Recovery is a journey of transformation, where each step forward is a reflection of your commitment to growth and self-improvement. Celebrate the progress you've made and the resilience you've shown, allowing these achievements to shape your self-image.

Mindfulness can be a valuable tool in addressing residual shame. By staying present in the moment, you can avoid ruminating on past mistakes or fearing judgment from others. Mindfulness helps you observe your thoughts and feelings without becoming overwhelmed by them, creating space for self-compassion and clarity. It reminds you that your worth is not tied to your past but exists in the here and now.

As you embrace a life free from shame, focus on cultivating a sense of gratitude for your journey. Recovery is not just about what you've overcome but also about the opportunities and insights it has provided. Reflect on the strength you've discovered within yourself, the relationships you've deepened, and the possibilities that lie ahead. Gratitude shifts your perspective from dwelling on what was lost to appreciating what you've gained.

Finally, living without shame is about accepting yourself fully, including the challenges you've faced. Your journey is part of your story, but it does not define your future. By embracing your worth and rejecting stigma, you create space for a life of authenticity, freedom, and fulfillment. The strength you've cultivated through recovery is a reminder that you are more than your past and that you have the power to shape a future aligned with your true self.

6.2. Staying Vigilant Against Relapse

Staying vigilant against relapse is a cornerstone of long-term recovery from addiction to pornography and masturbation. While significant progress is often made during the early stages of recovery, maintaining that progress requires ongoing awareness and intentionality. Relapse is not a sign of failure but a potential risk in the journey toward freedom, and understanding how to prevent it is crucial for sustaining the positive changes you've worked so hard to achieve.

The first step in staying vigilant is recognizing that recovery is a lifelong process. The habits and thought patterns associated with addiction don't disappear overnight; they require consistent effort to rewire. Relapse prevention begins with the acknowledgment that temptations and triggers may arise, even after extended periods of success. This awareness prepares you to face challenges with confidence rather than complacency, ensuring that you remain proactive in your recovery.

Identifying your personal triggers is essential for staying vigilant. Triggers can be external, such as specific environments, media, or social situations, or internal, like stress, boredom, or emotional discomfort. Reflect on the circumstances that have led to past challenges or setbacks, and consider how you can either avoid or prepare for them. For example, if certain times of day are particularly vulnerable, create a routine that fills those moments with engaging, positive activities. By understanding and addressing your triggers, you reduce their ability to derail your progress.

Establishing a daily routine that prioritizes self-care and well-being is another powerful tool for relapse prevention. A structured day leaves less room for idle moments that can lead to temptation. Incorporate practices like exercise, mindfulness, journaling, or pursuing hobbies to keep yourself focused and grounded. These activities not only occupy your time but also contribute to your overall mental and emotional resilience, making you less susceptible to urges.

Accountability is a vital component of staying vigilant. Sharing your recovery goals with a trusted friend, partner, or support group creates a sense of responsibility and provides encouragement during difficult times. Regular check-ins, whether in person or online, help you stay connected and committed to your journey. Knowing that others are aware of your efforts can reinforce your determination and remind you of the broader support network that is cheering you on.

Maintaining vigilance also involves practicing emotional awareness and regulation. Addiction often serves as a way to cope with uncomfortable emotions, such as stress, loneliness, or frustration. By developing healthy coping mechanisms and staying attuned to your feelings, you can address these emotions before they escalate into urges. Techniques like mindfulness, deep breathing, or talking with a trusted confidant can help you navigate emotional challenges without resorting to old habits.

One of the most effective ways to prevent relapse is to keep your recovery goals front and center. Remind yourself regularly why you chose to break free from addiction and what you've gained through your efforts. Write down your motivations and revisit them during moments of doubt or temptation. This practice reinforces your commitment and helps you stay focused on the bigger picture of your recovery journey.

Building a strong support system is also crucial for staying vigilant. Surround yourself with people who encourage your growth and share your values. These relationships provide a buffer against isolation and serve as a source of strength during challenging times. Whether it's friends, family members, or members of a recovery group, having a community that supports your well-being makes it easier to stay on track.

Developing a plan for how to handle setbacks is another essential part of vigilance. Despite your best efforts, challenges may arise, and knowing how to respond can make all the difference. If you find yourself facing a slip or relapse, avoid falling into the trap of shame or self-blame. Instead, view the setback as an opportunity to learn and grow. Reflect on what triggered the relapse, identify what could be done differently next time, and recommit to your recovery plan. This resilience ensures that a temporary misstep doesn't derail your long-term progress.

Revisiting and refining your recovery strategies over time is also important. As you grow and evolve, new challenges may emerge, requiring you to adapt your approach. Regularly assess what is working well and where adjustments might be needed. This ongoing reflection keeps your recovery dynamic and responsive to your changing needs.

Finally, celebrate your successes, no matter how small. Recovery is a journey of progress, and each day free from addiction is an achievement worth acknowledging. These celebrations reinforce your belief in your ability to maintain freedom and remind you of the rewards of your efforts. Whether it's treating yourself to something special, sharing your progress with a loved one, or simply taking a moment to reflect on your growth, these acts of recognition motivate you to keep moving forward.

Staying vigilant against relapse is about embracing the ongoing nature of recovery with intention and self-compassion. It's about recognizing that challenges are part of the journey and equipping yourself with the tools and mindset to navigate them successfully. By remaining proactive, connected, and reflective, you ensure that the progress you've made becomes the foundation for a life of freedom, balance, and fulfillment. Each moment of vigilance is a step toward reinforcing the positive changes you've created and embracing the limitless possibilities of your future.

6.3. Developing a Positive Relationship with Sexuality

Developing a positive relationship with sexuality is a crucial step in maintaining long-term recovery from addiction to pornography and masturbation. Addiction often distorts perceptions of sexuality, reducing it to a transactional or purely physical experience while neglecting its deeper emotional and relational aspects. Rebuilding your understanding of sexuality as a healthy, fulfilling, and integrated part of your life is not only possible but also essential for sustaining freedom and personal growth.

A positive relationship with sexuality begins with self-acceptance and self-awareness. Addiction can often leave individuals feeling ashamed or disconnected from their sexual identity. The first step in redefining your relationship with sexuality is to let go of shame and recognize that sexuality is a natural and valuable part of being human. It's not something to be feared or suppressed but embraced in a way that aligns with your values and personal goals.

Understanding the broader dimensions of sexuality is key to this transformation. True sexual well-being encompasses emotional intimacy, trust, and mutual respect. It's about creating connections—both with yourself and with others—that are meaningful, consensual, and enriching. Moving away from the superficial representations often portrayed in pornography allows you to explore the profound ways in which sexuality can deepen relationships and enhance your life.

One way to foster a healthier perspective on sexuality is by educating yourself. Reading about sexual health, relationships, and intimacy can help you broaden your understanding and dispel misconceptions. Resources written by experts in sexology or relational psychology provide valuable insights into how sexuality intersects with emotional, physical, and mental well-being. This knowledge empowers you to approach your sexuality with confidence and intention.

Mindfulness can also play a significant role in developing a positive relationship with sexuality. Mindfulness encourages you to stay present, fully experiencing the sensations and emotions that arise during moments of intimacy. This practice helps you reconnect with your body and mind in a way that is free from judgment or distraction. It shifts the focus away from external expectations or comparisons, allowing you to embrace the uniqueness of your own experiences.

For those in a romantic relationship, open communication with your partner is essential. Addiction can sometimes create barriers to intimacy or trust, and rebuilding these aspects of your relationship requires honesty and vulnerability. Share your feelings, fears, and desires with your partner, and invite them to do the same. These conversations foster a deeper connection and help you align your expectations and boundaries. If discussing these topics feels challenging, consider seeking the guidance of a therapist or counselor to navigate these conversations together.

Setting boundaries around sexual behavior is another important aspect of creating a healthier relationship with sexuality. Reflect on what behaviors align with your values and contribute to your well-being. For example, you might establish boundaries around when and how you engage with sexual content or decide to focus on cultivating intimacy in ways that prioritize connection and mutual respect. These boundaries are not about restriction but about creating a framework that supports your growth and self-respect.

For those who are not currently in a romantic relationship, developing a positive relationship with sexuality might involve exploring how you view yourself and your needs. Take time to reflect on your values and what sexuality means to you outside the context of addiction. Embrace the opportunity to redefine your sexual identity in a way that feels empowering and aligned with your goals.

Engaging in activities that promote physical and emotional well-being can also support a healthier approach to sexuality. Regular exercise, mindfulness practices, and self-care routines help you feel more connected to your body and emotions, enhancing your overall sense of self-worth. When you feel confident and balanced in other areas of your life, it becomes easier to approach your sexuality with positivity and intention.

Understanding the role of vulnerability in sexuality is another important step. True intimacy often requires the courage to be seen and accepted as you are, without pretense or performance. Embracing vulnerability allows you to form deeper, more authentic connections with others and to experience sexuality as an expression of trust and mutual respect. This shift moves away from the impersonal dynamics of addiction and toward a richer, more meaningful experience.

Lastly, give yourself permission to approach sexuality with curiosity and patience. Recovery is a journey of self-discovery, and rebuilding your relationship with sexuality takes time. Allow yourself to explore what feels right for you, and be open to learning and growing along the way. Celebrate the progress you make and recognize that every step you take is a testament to your commitment to living a balanced and fulfilling life.

Developing a positive relationship with sexuality is about more than overcoming addiction—it's about embracing your identity as a whole person. It's about seeing sexuality not as a source of shame or struggle but as a natural, beautiful part of who you are. By cultivating this relationship with intention and care, you create a foundation for lasting freedom, meaningful connections, and a life that reflects your values and aspirations.

6.4. How to Seek Help When Needed

Seeking help when needed is a vital part of sustaining long-term recovery from addiction to pornography and masturbation. Recovery is not a solitary journey; it's a process that often benefits from the insights, support, and guidance of others. Recognizing when you need help—and having the courage to reach out—is a sign of strength, not weakness. It shows a commitment to your well-being and a willingness to do whatever it takes to stay on the path of growth and healing.

The need for help can arise at different stages of recovery and for various reasons. You might encounter unexpected challenges, feel overwhelmed by emotions, or struggle to stay consistent with the habits you've established. Relapse, feelings of stagnation, or uncertainty about the next steps can also signal the need for external support. Acknowledging these moments is the first step in ensuring they don't derail your progress.

There are many forms of help available, ranging from professional support to peer-based communities. One of the most effective resources for recovery is therapy. A licensed therapist, particularly one specializing in addiction or sexual health, can provide a safe and confidential space to explore your thoughts, emotions, and behaviors. Therapists are trained to help you identify patterns, develop coping strategies, and address underlying issues that may contribute to addictive behavior. Whether you seek therapy during moments of crisis or as a proactive step, it can be a transformative tool in your recovery journey.

Group therapy or support groups are another invaluable resource. Groups like Sex Addicts Anonymous (SAA) or NoFap offer a community of individuals who understand the struggles you're facing and share similar goals. These groups provide not only practical advice but also a sense of belonging and accountability. Sharing your experiences in a supportive environment can reduce feelings of isolation and remind you that you are not alone in your challenges or successes.

For those who prefer a more self-directed approach, books, online courses, and recovery apps can offer guidance and structure. Resources like these allow you to learn at your own pace while providing tools to navigate specific aspects of recovery. However, it's important to supplement self-help efforts with opportunities for human connection, as interaction and accountability are often crucial for lasting change.

Friends and family can also be a source of help, though it's essential to choose the right individuals to share your journey with. Seek out those who are understanding, nonjudgmental, and supportive of your recovery goals. Having someone you trust to confide in during moments of doubt or temptation can make a significant difference. These trusted individuals can provide perspective, encouragement, and a reminder of your resilience and progress.

If you're in a romantic relationship, your partner can play a pivotal role in supporting your recovery. Open and honest communication about your struggles and goals creates a foundation of trust and understanding. Be mindful, however, of the balance between seeking support and relying too heavily on your partner for emotional stability. Your recovery is ultimately your responsibility, and while their encouragement is valuable, maintaining independence in your efforts is crucial.

In some cases, seeking help may involve addressing related challenges that impact your recovery. For example, unresolved trauma, anxiety, or depression can fuel addictive behaviors, making it difficult to sustain progress. Working with a mental health professional to address these issues not only supports your overall well-being but also strengthens your ability to maintain freedom from addiction.

Reaching out for help doesn't have to wait until a crisis arises. Being proactive about seeking guidance and building a support network ensures that you have resources in place when challenges occur. Regular check-ins with a therapist, attendance at support groups, or even periodic conversations with trusted friends can help you stay grounded and focused on your goals.

Overcoming the fear of seeking help is often a hurdle in itself. Stigma, shame, or the belief that you should handle everything on your own can discourage you from reaching out. Remember that seeking help is a normal and necessary part of growth. Everyone needs support at different points in life, and asking for it shows wisdom and self-awareness. It demonstrates your commitment to prioritizing your well-being and taking control of your future.

When seeking help, be open to the idea that your needs may evolve over time. What works for you at one stage of recovery might not be as effective later on, and that's okay. Stay curious and adaptable, exploring new resources and approaches as needed. Recovery is a dynamic process, and your willingness to seek help when needed ensures that you remain equipped to navigate its complexities.

Finally, seeking help is an act of self-respect and care. It's a recognition that you deserve support and that your journey toward freedom and fulfillment is worth every effort. By surrounding yourself with the tools, people, and resources that uplift you, you create a solid foundation for maintaining long-term recovery and embracing the life you are building. Asking for help is not just a step in recovery—it's a powerful declaration of your commitment to your growth, health, and happiness.

6.5. Inspiring Others Through Your Journey

Inspiring others through your journey is a powerful way to solidify your recovery while making a meaningful impact on those around you. Sharing your experiences, insights, and lessons not only helps others who may be struggling but also deepens your own commitment to a life of growth and freedom. By transforming your challenges into a source of inspiration, you create a legacy of resilience, compassion, and empowerment that extends beyond your personal journey.

One of the most impactful ways to inspire others is by being open about your recovery. Addiction often thrives in secrecy, and sharing your story breaks the silence that keeps many people from seeking help. When you speak openly about your struggles and successes, you normalize the conversation around addiction and recovery, showing others that it's possible to overcome challenges and reclaim control over their lives. Your honesty and vulnerability can be a beacon of hope for those who feel isolated or ashamed.

Inspiring others doesn't necessarily mean sharing every detail of your journey. You can tailor your openness to the context and your comfort level. Whether it's a heartfelt conversation with a friend, a post on social media, or participation in a support group, the act of sharing even small parts of your experience can have a profound impact. Your authenticity and willingness to speak out demonstrate that recovery is achievable and worth pursuing.

Mentorship is another meaningful way to inspire others. As someone who has navigated the path of recovery, you have valuable insights and experiences that can guide and encourage those just starting their journey. Mentorship can take many forms, from offering advice to someone in a recovery group to simply being a supportive friend or confidant. By sharing your knowledge and providing a listening ear, you help others find the strength and direction they need to overcome their struggles.

For those who feel comfortable, public advocacy is a powerful way to inspire change on a broader scale. Addiction to pornography and masturbation is often misunderstood or stigmatized, and raising awareness helps to challenge these misconceptions. Writing articles, speaking at events, or contributing to community discussions allows you to share your perspective and promote a deeper understanding of recovery. Your voice can contribute to a culture of empathy and support, making it easier for others to seek help without fear of judgment.

Engaging in creative outlets is another way to inspire others through your journey. Writing, art, music, or film can convey your experiences and emotions in a way that resonates deeply with others. These mediums allow you to express the complexities of recovery, offering insight and hope to those who may be struggling. Creativity not only inspires others but also serves as a therapeutic outlet for reflecting on your growth and celebrating your progress.

Inspiring others doesn't always require grand gestures. Small acts of kindness and encouragement can make a significant difference in someone's life. Offering words of support, sharing a helpful resource, or simply being present during a difficult moment demonstrates the power of connection and compassion. These acts create ripples of positivity that extend far beyond the immediate interaction.

As you inspire others, it's important to maintain healthy boundaries and prioritize your own well-being. While sharing your story and supporting others can be incredibly rewarding, it's essential to ensure that these efforts don't overwhelm or distract you from your own recovery. Balance is key—contribute in ways that feel sustainable and affirming, and don't hesitate to step back if needed.

Inspiring others through your journey also reinforces your own recovery. Each time you share your story or offer support, you reaffirm your commitment to the values and goals that have guided your transformation. These interactions remind you of how far you've come and reinforce the importance of staying on the path you've chosen. The act of helping others often deepens your sense of purpose and fulfillment, creating a cycle of positive reinforcement.

Finally, inspiring others is about creating a legacy of hope and empowerment. Your journey is a testament to the strength of the human spirit and the possibility of change. By sharing that journey, you contribute to a world where addiction is met with understanding and support, and recovery is seen as a courageous and achievable goal. Each person you inspire becomes part of this legacy, carrying forward the lessons and encouragement they've received to help others in turn.

Inspiring others is a way of giving back—to the community, to those who have supported you, and to the person you've become. It's a celebration of your growth and a reminder that the struggles you've faced have value, not just for yourself but for others who can learn from and be uplifted by your experiences. Through your story, you have the power to ignite hope, foster connection, and make a lasting difference in the lives of others.

6.6. A New Chapter: Embracing Freedom

Embracing a new chapter in life after addiction is about stepping fully into the freedom, possibility, and self-discovery that recovery offers. This final stage of your journey is not just about what you've overcome but about who you are becoming. It's a celebration of your growth, a commitment to living authentically, and an opportunity to shape a future that aligns with your deepest values and aspirations.

The decision to embrace a new chapter begins with letting go of the past. Addiction may have left behind memories of struggle, moments of regret, or lingering doubts, but your recovery has shown that you are not defined by those experiences. They are part of your story, but they do not dictate your future. Moving forward involves acknowledging the lessons you've learned and using them as a foundation for the life you want to create.

This new chapter is an invitation to explore the person you are today. Recovery has likely revealed strengths, passions, and desires that may have been overshadowed by addiction. Take time to reflect on who you are now—what excites you, what brings you joy, and what kind of life you want to build. These reflections help you reconnect with your authentic self and provide clarity for the path ahead.

Embracing this chapter also involves continuing to nurture the habits and practices that have supported your recovery. The routines, relationships, and strategies you've developed are not just tools for overcoming addiction; they are building blocks for a fulfilling life. Whether it's mindfulness, physical activity, or pursuing hobbies, these practices remind you of the power of intentional living and reinforce the positive changes you've made.

Setting new goals is an exciting part of this process. These goals might involve career aspirations, personal development, relationships, or creative pursuits. Whatever they are, they provide a sense of direction and purpose, motivating you to keep growing and evolving. Break these goals into manageable steps, and celebrate each milestone along the way. These achievements remind you of your capabilities and affirm your ability to create a life that reflects your dreams.

As you embrace this chapter, it's important to remain open to change and adaptability. Life is dynamic, and the journey of self-discovery is ongoing. Stay curious and willing to explore new opportunities, even if they feel outside your comfort zone. Each new experience is a chance to learn more about yourself and the world around you, deepening your understanding and expanding your horizons.

This stage of recovery also offers the opportunity to cultivate deeper connections with others. Whether it's strengthening existing relationships or forming new ones, these connections enrich your life and provide a sense of belonging. Be present and intentional in your interactions, focusing on building relationships that reflect mutual respect, trust, and support. These bonds remind you of the joy and fulfillment that come from authentic human connection.

Living in this new chapter means embracing the challenges as well as the triumphs. Recovery does not mean life will be free of difficulties, but it equips you with the tools and resilience to navigate them. Approach challenges with the same courage and determination that have guided your recovery, knowing that each obstacle is an opportunity for growth.

Gratitude is a powerful companion in this phase of your journey. Take time to reflect on the progress you've made, the support you've received, and the possibilities that lie ahead. Gratitude shifts your perspective from focusing on what was lost to appreciating what has been gained. It reminds you of the richness and potential of your life, encouraging you to approach each day with optimism and hope.

This chapter is also a chance to give back, whether by inspiring others through your story, supporting someone else's recovery, or contributing to your community in meaningful ways. Sharing the strength and insights you've gained enriches the lives of others while deepening your own sense of purpose. It's a reminder that the growth you've experienced has value not just for yourself but for the world around you.

Ultimately, embracing a new chapter is about honoring the journey you've taken and the person you've become. It's about living with intention, pursuing what matters most to you, and continuing to grow in ways that reflect your true self. This chapter is not the end of your story but the beginning of a life where you are free to explore, connect, and thrive.

As you move forward, carry with you the lessons, strength, and hope that have emerged from your recovery. Let them guide you as you build a life filled with meaning, joy, and authenticity. This new chapter is yours to write, and the possibilities are limitless. Embrace it fully, with confidence and an open heart, knowing that the best is yet to come.

Conclusion

Recovery is not just about breaking free from addiction—it's about reclaiming your life, rediscovering your worth, and embracing the limitless possibilities that lie ahead. As you reach the conclusion of this guide, it's important to take a moment to reflect on how far you've come. The courage it takes to face addiction, the commitment required to change, and the resilience needed to keep moving forward are all testaments to your strength and determination.

This journey has been one of growth and transformation, but it's not the end—it's the foundation for everything that comes next. The tools and strategies you've learned throughout this guide are now part of your daily life, empowering you to navigate challenges, build meaningful relationships, and continue growing as an individual. Each step you've taken, no matter how small, has brought you closer to the person you want to be.

As you move forward, remember that recovery is a dynamic process. Life will present new challenges, but the resilience and self-awareness you've cultivated will help you face them with confidence. Stay vigilant, practice self-compassion, and remain open to growth. Your journey doesn't require perfection—only persistence and a willingness to continue striving for a life that aligns with your values and aspirations.

Take pride in the progress you've made and the freedom you've achieved. Celebrate your successes, honor your efforts, and recognize the strength that brought you here. Your journey is not just about overcoming addiction; it's about reclaiming your identity, fostering connection, and creating a future filled with purpose and fulfillment.

You are not alone on this path. Others have walked it before you, and many more will follow in your footsteps. By sharing your story, offering support, or simply living authentically, you have the power to inspire others and contribute to a culture of understanding and compassion. Your recovery is not just a personal victory—it's a source of hope and encouragement for others who are seeking freedom.

As you close this chapter, let it be a reminder of what you've achieved and a motivation for what lies ahead. Embrace the possibilities, trust in your ability to grow, and hold onto the vision of the life you're building. This is not just the conclusion of a guide; it's the beginning of a life lived fully, authentically, and with intention.

The journey you've undertaken is a remarkable one, and it's a testament to your strength and determination. You've reclaimed your life—now it's time to live it to the fullest. The future is yours to shape, and the possibilities are endless. Embrace it with confidence, purpose, and the knowledge that you are capable of achieving great things.

Reflecting on Your Progress

Reflecting on your progress is a powerful and affirming exercise that allows you to fully appreciate the journey you've undertaken to overcome addiction to pornography and masturbation. Recovery is not just about the destination—it's about the growth, resilience, and self-discovery that occur along the way. Taking the time to acknowledge and reflect on how far you've come reinforces your sense of achievement, deepens your self-awareness, and motivates you to continue building the life you want.

Start by considering where you began. Think back to the moments when addiction felt overwhelming, when the idea of breaking free seemed distant or impossible. Remember the struggles you faced, the emotions you grappled with, and the patterns that kept you feeling stuck. Reflecting on these moments is not about revisiting pain but about recognizing the tremendous strength it took to move beyond them. Your journey began with a decision to change, and that choice was the first step toward reclaiming your life.

As you reflect, take note of the tools and strategies you've adopted to support your recovery. Perhaps mindfulness helped you manage urges, or a consistent daily routine provided structure and stability. Maybe reaching out to a trusted friend or support group gave you the courage to keep going when things felt difficult. Each of these tools is a testament to your resourcefulness and willingness to embrace change. Recognizing what has worked for you not only highlights your progress but also provides a foundation for sustaining your freedom.

Consider the challenges you've faced along the way and how you responded to them. Recovery is rarely a linear path, and setbacks or moments of doubt are a natural part of the process. Reflect on how you navigated these moments—what you learned, how you adapted, and how you found the strength to keep moving forward. These challenges were not failures but opportunities to grow, and your ability to persevere through them is a reflection of your resilience.

Think about the positive changes you've experienced since beginning your recovery. These might include tangible milestones, such as reduced urges or a greater sense of control, as well as more subtle shifts, like improved emotional well-being, stronger relationships, or a renewed sense of purpose. Each of these changes is a victory, a sign of the transformation that recovery has brought into your life. Celebrate these wins, no matter how small they may seem, as they collectively represent the progress you've made.

Take a moment to reflect on how your sense of self has evolved. Addiction often distorts self-perception, creating feelings of shame or inadequacy. Through recovery, you've had the opportunity to reconnect with your true self, to rediscover your strengths, values, and aspirations. Reflect on the person you are becoming—someone who is courageous, self-aware, and committed to living authentically. Recognizing this growth fosters a deeper sense of self-respect and confidence.

As you reflect, it's also important to acknowledge the support you've received along the way. Recovery is a journey often enriched by the encouragement and understanding of others. Whether it was a friend, family member, therapist, or support group, these connections played a role in your progress. Take time to express gratitude for the people and resources that have supported you, as their contributions are part of the foundation upon which your recovery is built.

Reflection is not just about looking back—it's also about looking ahead. Use this time to consider how you want to build on the progress you've made. What goals do you have for the future? What aspects of your recovery would you like to strengthen or deepen? By identifying areas for continued growth, you create a sense of direction and purpose that keeps you moving forward.

Finally, be kind to yourself as you reflect. Recovery is a journey of effort and perseverance, and the fact that you've come this far is an accomplishment worth celebrating. Treat yourself with the compassion and understanding you deserve, recognizing that every step you've taken has brought you closer to a life of freedom and fulfillment.

Reflecting on your progress is a way of honoring your journey and the person you are becoming. It reminds you of the strength and determination you've shown, the lessons you've learned, and the possibilities that lie ahead. Take pride in how far you've come, and let that pride inspire you to keep growing, exploring, and embracing the life you're building. Each moment of reflection is a reminder of your resilience and a celebration of the remarkable progress you've made.

The Journey Ahead: Growth Beyond Addiction

The journey ahead after overcoming addiction to pornography and masturbation is filled with growth, self-discovery, and the boundless potential to build a life aligned with your values and aspirations. Recovery is not just about leaving something behind; it's about moving forward with intention, embracing your freedom, and continually evolving into the person you want to be. This stage of your journey is an opportunity to explore new possibilities, deepen your understanding of yourself, and create a future defined by purpose and fulfillment.

Growth beyond addiction begins with a mindset of curiosity and openness. Recovery has given you the tools to confront challenges and the resilience to overcome them. Now, you can use those same strengths to explore areas of your life that you may have neglected or overlooked. What dreams have you put on hold? What passions have you yet to pursue? Allow yourself to imagine a future that excites and inspires you, and take steps to make it a reality.

This phase of your journey is also about reinforcing the habits and practices that have supported your recovery. The routines, coping strategies, and mindfulness techniques you've developed are not just tools for overcoming addiction—they are the foundation for a balanced and meaningful life. By continuing to prioritize these practices, you maintain the structure and stability that empower you to navigate life's challenges with confidence.

As you grow beyond addiction, it's important to remain vigilant and self-aware. Freedom from addiction doesn't mean that challenges will disappear entirely, but it does mean that you are equipped to face them. Stay attuned to your triggers, emotions, and patterns, and address any vulnerabilities with the same intentionality that guided your recovery. Self-awareness is your compass, helping you stay aligned with your values and goals as you navigate the complexities of life.

Relationships play a vital role in the journey ahead. Recovery has likely deepened your understanding of connection and intimacy, and now is the time to nurture and expand these relationships. Whether it's strengthening bonds with loved ones, forming new friendships, or exploring romantic partnerships, prioritize connections that bring joy, support, and authenticity to your life. These relationships are a source of strength and inspiration, reminding you of the richness and meaning that come from genuine human connection.

This stage of your journey also offers the opportunity to redefine your relationship with yourself. Addiction often creates a distorted self-image, but recovery allows you to rediscover your worth and potential. Take time to celebrate the progress you've made and the qualities that make you unique. Embrace self-compassion and treat yourself with the kindness and respect you deserve. By cultivating a positive relationship with yourself, you create a strong foundation for continued growth and fulfillment.

Exploring new challenges and opportunities is a key aspect of growth beyond addiction. This might involve pursuing education or career goals, volunteering in your community, or developing skills in areas that interest you. These endeavors not only expand your horizons but also reinforce your sense of purpose and capability. Each new experience is a chance to learn, grow, and contribute, adding depth and meaning to your life.

Giving back is another powerful way to continue your growth. Sharing your journey, offering support to others, or raising awareness about addiction and recovery can create a ripple effect of positivity and hope. Your experiences have given you unique insights and strengths that can inspire and uplift those who are just beginning their own journeys. By contributing to the recovery community or advocating for greater understanding, you turn your challenges into a source of empowerment and change.

Spiritual or philosophical exploration can also play a significant role in the journey ahead. Recovery often prompts questions about purpose, meaning, and identity, and this phase of your life is an opportunity to explore those questions more deeply. Whether through meditation, faith practices, or personal reflection, connecting with something larger than yourself can provide a sense of grounding and direction that enriches your life.

Finally, embrace the idea that growth is an ongoing process. There is no finish line to recovery or self-improvement; rather, life is a continuous journey of learning and evolving. Approach each day with a sense of curiosity and gratitude, recognizing that every experience— whether joyful or challenging—is an opportunity to grow.

The journey ahead is yours to shape, and the possibilities are endless. You've already proven your strength, resilience, and commitment by overcoming addiction. Now, it's time to channel those qualities into creating a life that reflects your values, passions, and dreams. Embrace this chapter with confidence and an open heart, knowing that the best is yet to come. Growth beyond addiction is not just about leaving something behind—it's about stepping boldly into the future and fully embracing the person you are meant to be.

Resources for Continued Support

As you move forward in your journey of recovery and growth, having access to reliable resources for continued support is invaluable. Recovery doesn't end with breaking free from addiction—it's a dynamic process of ongoing learning, self-care, and personal development. Surrounding yourself with tools and communities that empower and encourage you will help you maintain the progress you've made and navigate any challenges that arise.

One of the most accessible resources for continued support is literature. Books on addiction recovery, personal growth, mindfulness, and emotional resilience can provide valuable insights and practical tools. Seek out works by experts in psychology, self-help, and relational health to deepen your understanding of the processes underlying addiction and recovery. These books can also serve as a source of inspiration, helping you stay motivated and focused on your goals.

Online platforms and forums dedicated to recovery are another valuable resource. Communities like Reddit's r/NoFap, Quit Porn Community, or specific addiction recovery websites offer spaces where individuals share their experiences, struggles, and successes. Engaging with these communities can provide a sense of belonging and accountability, as well as practical advice and encouragement from people who understand your journey.

Support groups, whether in person or virtual, offer a structured and empathetic environment for recovery. Groups like Sex Addicts Anonymous (SAA), Celebrate Recovery, or local addiction support organizations provide a safe space to share your experiences, learn from others, and build connections. These groups often follow established frameworks that promote personal accountability and growth, helping you stay committed to your recovery.

For those who prefer personalized guidance, therapy or counseling remains a cornerstone of continued support. A licensed therapist, particularly one specializing in addiction or sexual health, can provide tailored strategies for navigating challenges and maintaining your progress. Therapy also offers a confidential space to explore deeper emotional or relational issues that may emerge during your journey. Teletherapy platforms like BetterHelp or Talkspace make accessing professional support more convenient than ever.

Mindfulness and meditation apps are excellent tools for emotional regulation and self-awareness. Platforms like Calm, Headspace, or Insight Timer offer guided meditations, relaxation exercises, and mindfulness practices that can help you manage stress, stay grounded, and maintain a positive outlook. These practices not only support your recovery but also enhance your overall mental and emotional well-being.

Habit-tracking apps are another practical resource. Tools like Streaks, Habitica, or Done allow you to set and track goals, monitor your progress, and stay motivated. Whether you're focusing on abstinence, building new habits, or developing healthy routines, these apps help you maintain consistency and celebrate your achievements along the way.

Educational courses and workshops can also support your recovery and personal growth. Many online platforms, such as Coursera, Udemy, or Skillshare, offer courses on topics ranging from psychology and emotional intelligence to personal development and mindfulness. These learning opportunities not only expand your knowledge but also provide constructive ways to use your time and energy.

If spirituality is an important part of your life, connecting with faith-based resources or communities can provide comfort and direction. Many religious or spiritual organizations offer support groups, counseling services, or resources specifically tailored to individuals recovering from addiction. Exploring your spiritual beliefs and practices can also provide a sense of purpose and connection that reinforces your recovery.

Developing a network of trusted individuals—whether friends, family, mentors, or peers—remains one of the most vital resources for ongoing support. Surround yourself with people who uplift and encourage you, and don't hesitate to lean on them during moments of doubt or difficulty. Their presence reminds you that you're not alone and that your journey is one worth celebrating and supporting.

Finally, consider creating your own personalized toolkit for recovery. This might include a journal for reflection, a playlist of motivating music, quotes or affirmations that inspire you, or a list of activities that bring you joy and fulfillment. Having these resources at your fingertips provides a quick and effective way to recenter yourself whenever challenges arise.

Recovery is an ongoing process, and having access to the right resources ensures that you remain supported and empowered every step of the way. By utilizing these tools, communities, and practices, you not only strengthen your recovery but also create a foundation for a life of growth, connection, and fulfillment. Remember, seeking support is not a sign of weakness—it's a powerful commitment to your well-being and the future you're building.

Final Words of Encouragement

As you reach the final pages of this guide, take a moment to honor the incredible courage and determination that brought you here. Choosing to confront addiction and embark on a journey of recovery is no small feat—it requires strength, self-awareness, and a willingness to embrace change. You have taken significant steps to reclaim your life, and that is an achievement worth celebrating.

Recovery is not just about overcoming addiction; it's about rediscovering who you are, what you value, and what brings meaning to your life. It's about building a future that reflects your dreams and aspirations, free from the patterns that once held you back. Along this journey, you've proven that growth is possible and that you are capable of transforming even the most difficult challenges into opportunities for self-discovery and renewal.

Remember, recovery is a process, not a destination. There will be moments of triumph and moments of difficulty, but each step you take brings you closer to the life you envision for yourself. In those challenging moments, draw strength from the progress you've made, the tools you've acquired, and the support systems you've built. Every setback is an opportunity to learn, and every success is a testament to your resilience.

As you move forward, embrace the idea that your journey is uniquely yours. There is no single path to recovery, and your experiences, struggles, and victories are a part of what makes you who you are. Be kind to yourself, practice self-compassion, and trust in your ability to navigate whatever lies ahead. You have already overcome so much, and you are capable of achieving even more.

Let this guide serve as a reminder of your strength and as a companion for the road ahead. Whenever you need encouragement, revisit the lessons and insights you've gathered here. Let them inspire you to keep striving for a life that reflects your values, passions, and potential.

You are not alone on this journey. Others have walked this path before you, and many will follow in your footsteps. By sharing your story, offering support, or simply living authentically, you have the power to inspire and uplift others. Your recovery is not only a personal triumph but also a source of hope and encouragement for those who are still searching for their way.

The freedom you've gained through recovery is a gift—one that allows you to live with intention, pursue your dreams, and connect deeply with the people and experiences that matter most. Embrace this freedom, celebrate your progress, and continue moving forward with confidence and purpose.

You are capable. You are resilient. You are worthy of a life filled with joy, connection, and fulfillment. The journey ahead is yours to shape, and the possibilities are limitless. Take this moment to acknowledge all that you've accomplished and look forward to the future with hope and determination. Your best days are still to come.